THE ALLERGY EPIDEMIC

Susan Prescott is a Paediatric Allergist and Immunologist at the leading children's hospital in Perth, and a Winthrop Professor at the University of Western Australia. She established and continues to run a highly productive clinical and laboratory research group within the University School of Paediatrics and Child Health. Professor Prescott is internationally recognised for her research in the area of allergy and early immune development.

DR SUSAN
PRESCOTT

...

The
Allergy
Epidemic

...

*A Mystery
of Modern Life*

UWA PUBLISHING

First published in 2011 by
UWA Publishing
Crawley, Western Australia 6009
www.uwap.uwa.edu.au

UWAP is an imprint of UWA Publishing
a division of The University of Western Australia

THE UNIVERSITY OF
WESTERN AUSTRALIA
Achieve International Excellence

National Library of Australia
Cataloguing-in-Publication data:

Prescott, Susan L.
The allergy epidemic: a mystery of modern life / Susan L. Prescott
9781742582917 (pbk.)
Includes bibliographical references
Allergy
Allergy—Treatment
Allergy—Environmental aspects

Typeset by J & M Typesetting
Printed by Griffin Press

This book is for the countless millions who suffer
the many burdens of allergic diseases, and for all those
who are working so hard to solve the mystery of
this epidemic.

CONTENTS

CONTENTS

Contents

CONTENTS

PREFACE

Allergies have emerged as a major public health problem. This enormous rise in disease has been most apparent in developed countries, and nowhere is this 'epidemic' more evident than in Australia and New Zealand, which have among the highest prevalence of allergic disorders in the world. Published studies indicate that the prevalence of allergies is continuing to increase, with a doubling in the rate of hospital admissions for potentially life threatening, severe allergic food reactions (anaphylaxis) in Australia over the past decade. The impact is even greater on preschool children who have experienced a five-fold increase in serious food allergy. It is now concerning to see the same trends beginning to emerge in many developing regions of the world.

The burden of the allergy epidemic is felt at every level. The personal impact and social costs are growing and the mounting economic costs are unparalleled. In a report published by Access Economics and the Australasian Society of Clinical Immunology and Allergy (ASCIA) it was estimated that the financial cost of allergies in Australia was $7.8 billion in 2007; and other developed countries are showing similar trends. This report also emphasised that raising awareness of allergies is an important factor in facilitating the early recognition and control of allergic disease.

We therefore commend Professor Susan Prescott in publishing this important book, which we believe will raise awareness of allergies by providing current, accurate and evidence-based information in a language that a lay person can understand.

Associate Professor Jo Douglass
President
Australian Society of Clinical Immunology
and Allergy

Associate Professor Richard Loh
President Elect
Australian Society of Clinical Immunology
and Allergy

FOREWORD

Allergy is one of the most common non-infectious diseases. The global increase in this disease is unprecedented, it affects all societies and brings with it vast personal, social and economic costs. The greatest burden of this 'epidemic' is borne by young children, who account for the most dramatic increase in disease. Already, about 30–40 per cent of the world's population is affected by one or more allergic conditions, including food allergies, eczema, allergic rhinitis and asthma. As the younger generations reach adulthood, the burden of allergic diseases is expected to increase even more. Many of these conditions can be serious and life threatening. It is therefore very important that allergy is recognised as a major public health problem and that continuous efforts are made towards its prevention and optimal treatment.

Promoting public awareness is an essential part of this process, and that is exactly what Professor Susan Prescott does in *The Allergy Epidemic: A Mystery of Modern Life*. In a time of uncertainty and confusion, she provides much needed clarity and hope, as she tells the fascinating yet serious story of allergy in the modern world. Not only does she describe and explain each allergic disease and its treatment, she also delves into the intriguing story that lies behind the epidemic rise in immune diseases and explains how and why this may be happening. She provides insights and information as she takes her readers into the world of the immune system in a way that captures the imagination and makes a very complex area of medical science immediate and accessible. At the cutting edge she explains the very latest research, and introduces important concepts that underpin many modern diseases including the new fields of 'developmental origins' and 'epigenetics', which are changing the way we understand the effects of modern environmental changes on our immune systems. Research in all these areas may provide new answers and solutions to the mystery of the allergy epidemic.

An allergy specialist and a pediatrician, Susan Prescott is also a leading research scientist, internationally recognised and highly regarded for her research into the developing immune system and how this system gets 'sidetracked' in allergic disease. She is also at the forefront of efforts to understand the environmental factors that are driving this epidemic, including approaches that might help reverse this through prevention strategies early in life.

The Allergy Epidemic coincides with another very important initiative: the release of the first ever, international *WAO White Book on Allergy*, published by the World Allergy Organization (WAO). The WAO *White Book on Allergy* targets governments and health care policy makers of the world, and makes high-level recommendations to address this growing international crisis. A key recommendation of the WAO *White Book on Allergy* is to 'increase public awareness of allergic diseases and their prevention'. In the light of this, Susan Prescott's highly accessible book on this central mystery of our modern life is a relevant and logical companion to the core objectives of the *White Book*.

Professor Ruby Pawankar,
MD PhD FAAAAI
President Elect
World Allergy Organization

1

In the trenches

We have never been so busy. I arrive to see the allergy clinic waiting room as overcrowded as usual. Brimming with children. Some scared, some screaming, some just bored. All ages. All with serious allergies. There are record numbers of new referrals. Our lists are so long that many have been waiting over a year for their appointment. And they just keep coming. We overbook them. We do extra clinics. But still we can't keep up.

There is no better place to see first-hand evidence of the allergy epidemic.

I momentarily close my door on the chaos to review my first chart. And I smile. I have known Ben since he was a small baby when he had a life-threatening reaction to cow's milk. He only had a mouthful. Karen, his mother was completely bewildered as her six-month-old son reacted almost instantly before her eyes. His lips swelled. His eyes swelled so much, he could hardly open them. A blotchy rash spread over most of his body and he started coughing and gasping for breath. Although panic stricken, Karen still had the presence of mind to call the ambulance. She had never been so relieved as when the paramedics came bursting through her door. Ben received a life-saving dose of adrenaline and Karen watched, amazed, as his symptoms settled almost as quickly as they had started. She had never heard of an 'anaphylactic' reaction before, but now she had first-hand experience.

That was thirteen years ago and I have been seeing Ben every year since. I call his name across the bedlam. It takes several attempts before they hear me. Then I see a strapping teenager, with his mother and younger sister Amy in tow, fighting their way across a floor strewn with toys and toddlers. As they settle themselves in the quiet of my consulting room, Karen presents some home-baked cakes. She proudly announces that they are made without eggs, dairy or nuts, for me to share with the other doctors in our tea break.

I take them gratefully, but don't tell her that we rarely have time for a break together these days. We are an all-girl team today. Each of us working behind a door in the long row of consulting rooms that surround the large clinic waiting room. Although I can't remember the last time we all sat down together for a tea-break, we still regularly drop into each other's rooms to discuss our more difficult and puzzling patients. And there seem to be more and more of those.

Things have changed so much, even since Ben first developed his allergies. Back in 1995, when I first started working in the allergy clinic, food allergies were already becoming common, but still nothing like they are now. And although some allergies like peanut and shellfish often persisted into adulthood, most other common forms of food allergy, like egg and milk allergy, were almost always transient. So, when I first met them, I confidently told Karen that Ben's milk allergy would likely be gone by the time he reached school age. That might have been the case then, but I have since had to eat those words more times than I care to remember. Not only are these food allergies becoming more common, they also seem to be becoming more persistent.

With each passing year Karen would wait expectantly to see the results of Ben's latest allergy tests. And each time my heart would sink as I prepared to disappoint her again. I am glad to say that many of our patients do still outgrow their egg and dairy allergies, but with the growing number of people who don't, we are now more cautious with our predictions!

Ben and his family have not had an easy journey. It was not long before he also developed an allergy to egg. And then peanuts. The level of vigilance needed while buying, preparing and eating food is very difficult, time-consuming and stressful, because the consequence of a mistake can be life threatening. And yet, like so many others, Karen and her family have taken this in their stride. It becomes a way of life.

Today we are checking that Ben is learning to take more responsibility for his own diet. We will update his adrenaline auto-injectors and make sure he knows how to use them himself. The teenage years can bring new challenges. Ben is very good but he still refuses to wear the medical alert bracelet, which warns of his allergies.

Even though Ben's allergies seem to be here to stay, we have never given up hope. So, once again, I key the computer to see the results of the blood tests he had last week. I look down the list of his allergic antibody levels to egg, milk and peanut. None of us is optimistic, but as always, there is an air of expectancy. Amy is just as interested, as everyone in the family is affected by Ben's restrictive diet. They are all watching my face and I try not to give too much away.

Just at that moment, there is a knock at the door, which opens before I can even answer. With an apologetic look, Terri, the allergy nurse, calmly announces that I am needed urgently in the treatment room. One of the food challenge patients is going into anaphylaxis.

Karen and Ben need no explanations for my hasty departure. Karen's look of understanding says it all, and reflects the memory of her own experience many years before. I arrive in the treatment room to find the situation already well in hand. Val, the nurse specialist has already given an injection of adrenaline and the junior doctor is monitoring the recovery of a two year old girl, Chloe. Another nurse is consoling Chloe's mother Madeleine, who is quietly in tears. Chloe also has milk allergy, but her recent allergy tests had shown such promising improvement; down to a level where we all felt it was worth trying a test feed or a 'food challenge' to see if she might be growing out of it. Madeleine had been very keen to try this. But, although Chloe has had more milk than she ever had before, she is clearly not ready yet.

We always do food challenges very slowly, starting with tiny amounts, so we can detect any reaction early. Chloe had been doing well, but on her third increment symptoms started to develop. First came the red blotchy rash. Then her eyes and nose started streaming. While these symptoms are not serious, the cough was the first sign that this might be evolving into anaphylaxis. The adrenaline, which was ready just in case, was given without delay. Red faced, but now settled, Chloe is looking happier than Madeleine. With everyone's heart rate returning to normal, I reassure Madeleine and arrange to see them momentarily, after I have finished seeing Ben.

Satisfied that all is well, I make my way back to where Karen, Ben and Amy are waiting patiently. Back in front of my computer screen, I re-inspect Ben's numbers. As expected, Ben's peanut antibodies are still so high they are above the laboratory's detection scale. No one is surprised, but there is still disappointment. But then I happily add some good news: that the milk and egg levels are looking better than ever. Finally, we may be able to strike these two foods off Ben's avoidance list. But first he will have to go through two food challenges, and after avoiding certain foods for so long, this can be quite a psychological obstacle.

No one speaks. This is a moment that they have all been waiting for. But Ben looks uncertain. Karen stunned. She quickly recovers and turns to Ben saying that she thinks this is great news. Trying to sound convincing, she tells him that she thinks that the challenges are worth trying and that this is the only way to find out. Life would be so much easier if they didn't have to avoid milk and eggs.

Ben still looks unsure, and I spend some time explaining the challenge procedure: how we do this gradually, starting with only a rub of food on the lip, and that we stop if there is any sign of a reaction, adrenaline always at the ready. I also explain that he will have plenty of time to think about it, because the waiting time for challenges is at least six months now. This seems to satisfy Ben, who gives the okay to start the paperwork and the bookings. In the meantime he actually seems relieved to continue with the avoidance diet that he has become so used to.

If the challenges go well, that might leave only peanut. And I have more good news on that front too.

They have heard there may be a cure for peanut allergy on the horizon and they want to know more about it. I begin to explain that there are new research trials under way using oral immunotherapy (OIT), aimed at potentially curing peanut allergy; how they are enrolling patients just like Ben, with very high allergic antibody levels and a history of anaphylaxis (Chapter 11). By starting with very tiny amounts of peanut and gradually building up the amount over weeks and months, the immune systems 'learn' to tolerate peanut and the patient can eventually cope with a sizeable portion each day. But this can be very dangerous and most children have reactions along the way. The aim of OIT is to change the underlying immune responses. This is quite different from the oral challenge, which is a short term 'test' of allergy that does not continue for long enough to change the immune responses to the food. Understandably, these procedures are only done under strict medical supervision because of the potential for life-threatening reactions. Even so, in studies done so far, many children eventually tolerate peanut as a regular part of their diet. The same technique has been used for other foods, such as milk and egg. At the moment this is still in the 'experimental stages' until the safest and most effective methods have been determined. It is not yet clear how long the effects will last, and how this may vary between children. With many unanswered questions, it will be some years before this may become available to patients in everyday practice. Even then, it won't be suitable for all patients with food allergy. Nonetheless, this provides a future hope that we could not offer before.

Ben is tuning out by now, and the idea of eating peanuts is too much to contemplate. I suspect he is grateful that this will not be any time soon.

Although the new 'oral immunotherapy' treatments are the first hope of a real cure for food allergy, they will create new difficulties in the clinic. In their current experimental form, they are very labour-intensive and require extended periods of medical observation. Most hospital clinics barely have the resources to cope with their current services. At the moment, none of us can imagine the logistics of how these treatments can be delivered to the thousands of children who could benefit. Still, with so many families affected by persistent food allergies, it is good to finally provide some light at the end of the tunnel, even if we are not yet sure how we will overcome the logistics of doing so.

It is something special to see the new hope in Karen's eyes. With a spring in my step, I see them back to the waiting area. Ben finally cracks a smile as he turns around to say goodbye.

By now Madeleine is also back in the waiting room, still looking shell-shocked, but much calmer. And Chloe is playing as though nothing has happened. When I call them in to my waiting room Chloe has a change of heart and starts screaming, clearly worried that we are about to do something else unpleasant. Struggling to be heard, we spend a few minutes going through Chloe's allergy management plan. She clearly needs to avoid all dairy products for a while yet. But unlike Ben, the early and progressive drop in her allergic antibody levels to milk still holds some promise that she will eventually grow out of it. And she has no signs of other food allergies. This might be because we have made sure that she started eating most other 'allergenic' foods, like peanut butter, regularly as early as possible. It initially took some convincing for Madeleine to do this because of the well-known previous approach of avoiding these foods in the hope of preventing new allergies. However, since new studies have suggested that avoidance is not effective, we now recommend that allergenic foods are included in the weaning diet without any specific avoidance (see Chapter 9).

Madeleine is convinced it was worth it. Now that Chloe has virtually all common foods as part of her regular diet, it is unlikely that she will develop allergies to any of them. Her immune system has already 'learned' to tolerate them. She remains at risk of other kinds of allergic diseases, like asthma and rhinitis as she gets older, but once the milk allergy is outgrown she should be free of any food allergies.

Like so many parents, Madeleine is still full of questions:

- Why did Chloe develop food allergy when no one else in the family has food allergy?
- What went wrong with her immune system to cause this?
- Is it genetic?
- Why are allergies on the increase?
- Are there factors in the environment that are causing this?
- Could we have done anything to prevent this?

She has her own theories. Most parents do. Many are convinced the modern environment is to blame. Some blame unseen toxins in the modern world, some blame antibiotics and cleaner living, and some blame more processed refined diets. And there is probably truth to all of these ideas.

Helpless to explain our current scientific ideas about these complex issues in the remaining moments we have left, I feel guilty in my cursory and superficial attempts. All I can do is agree wholeheartedly that our modern lifestyle is a driving force behind the allergy epidemic.

And I start to question what I am doing. I am a clinician, but I am also a researcher, a scientist and a teacher. I travel the world as an expert in this field, giving lectures and talking to many other international experts. I write research papers, editorials, opinion papers and book chapters. All for other clinicians and scientists. Suddenly it seems illogical and extraordinary that I am not bringing my roles together more; teaching and writing for the very people who ask these questions of us every day in the clinic, the people who are actually living the effects of the allergy crisis on a daily basis.

There have been so many fascinating and exciting developments in our understanding of the immune system, the environment, our genes and how these all interact to produce the rise in many modern diseases. We might not have all the answers yet, but the rate of recent discovery is cause for great optimism. The problem is that there is still so much misinformation and misconception out there. It is no wonder that many parents and patients get confused. We are so busy dealing with the effects of the epidemic that we often don't take the time to explain what we know about it. Unless experts at the cutting edge of research take the time to communicate more of these things to the people who really want to know, none of this will get any clearer.

This small revelation dawns on me in the few moments that it takes to see Madeleine and Chloe back to the waiting area. I pick up the next chart, ready for the next story. And as I look at the sea of faces and the many charts piled up in my box, I feel a new sense of purpose.

2

The making of an allergist

After my clinic I head back to my University office on the other side of the Children's Hospital campus to prepare for a teaching session. Another part of my role as a University Professor is to teach the next generation of doctors. The medical students rotate through our hospital to study Paediatrics and Child Health and this is an opportunity to teach them about the common allergies that begin in childhood, such as eczema, food allergy, rhinitis ('hay fever') and asthma. As I collect my teaching materials, I hear the boisterous students returning from the wards for our classroom session. We have about thirty students on this rotation and the seminar room is packed and raucous when I arrive. Standing in front of the next generation of doctors, I remember sitting in those same classroom chairs, with my own unformed, innocent enthusiasm.

• • •

I suppose we all have moments when we zone out and suddenly wonder: how the hell did I get here? As a very young child I had many high ambitions, and these changed daily: I wanted to be a teacher, a writer, a performer, a doctor, a leader, an artist, an actor, a scientist. Anything seemed possible. Only when I consider it from where I am now do I see that, in strangeness, I do indeed do all of these things. It might seem more by accident than by design, but I suspect that even after they slip into our subconscious, untamed childhood dreams have more power than we realise. There are certainly things I never planned to do, and might have even shied away from; I never thought to be a fundraiser, an account manager or a peace maker but somehow these roles are always on my 'to do' list as well. But none of this was clear to me at sixteen when I finished high school.

Poised on the threshold of an uncertain future, I wanted to make a difference on any scale that had meaning. It was exciting to have an entirely blank slate in front of me. I felt I could put anything on it, but I hesitated to make a commitment. Rather than find uncertainty daunting, I loved the feeling of an open horizon of endless possibilities. That was my problem. I did not want to narrow my horizons by making choices. At least that was my excuse. I *liked* having possibility, uncertainty. A strong sense of purpose, yet undefined; a wanting without shape. My naïve enthusiasm had grown under the nurturing care of my new-age parents, who also went to great lengths not to taint, bias or influence my choices in any way.

It was my more traditional grandparents that gave focus to my passion. My grandmother, Monica, was one of the very few women to study medicine in the 1930s. From a family of adventurers, explorers and missionaries, she had taken inspiration from her father who believed that 'travel was the best education'. As one of the first protestant missionaries to Peru in the early 1900s, he had travelled the dangerous mountain passes of the Andes by mule to provide basic medical care. His exotic tales and sometimes hair-raising journeys became bedtime stories for Monica and her sister throughout their childhood. They revelled in his adventures, inspired to believe that anything was possible. Although they were very poor, they always lived by the motto that 'where there is a will, there is a way', and Monica set her heart on medicine from an early age. Following in her father's footsteps, she sailed out to China as a medical missionary as soon as she finished medical school in 1937, just as war was breaking out.

I first came to hear Monica's stories of working as a doctor in Japanese-occupied China when I was sixteen. Just finished high school, still uncertain and waiting for my exam results, Monica announced that she would like to honour her father's belief that 'travel is the best education' and take me to Europe for several months as her travelling companion. It was during those travels that I got to know her more and my own plans to study medicine were set, not to mention my own love of travel. I was enthralled by her passion and how she had always known she wanted to study medicine and become a medical missionary. Because her family had been so poor and scholarships were very difficult to get, she had to be creative. She found a scholarship given to somebody who didn't drink, didn't smoke, and went to church regularly, and joked that she might have been the only eligible candidate. Monica then seemed to approach her medical training with much the same spirit of enthusiasm and fearlessness as she approached every other aspect of her life. There was never any sense that she might be at all intimidated by the establishment, or by the social class, gender or intelligence of her mainly male peers. As one of so few women, I once asked her if she experienced any prejudice or intimidation. I was surprised by her answer. She said that it just never occurred to her that this might be an issue, and because she did not make it an issue she did not experience it. She delighted in the company of her male colleagues and they delighted in hers. They all just 'got on with it'. This is a philosophy that I have tried to hold onto in my own career.

Monica's eyes always shone when she recalled her days of medicine, and I think this played a large part in my decision. I am equally determined when I set my goals but I tend to follow my heart more than my head when opportunities arise. Listening to

Monica there came a moment when I suddenly just knew in my heart that medicine was for me too. When I look back I cannot imagine doing anything else.

She told me of how she had seen medicine transform the world in a very short span of years. It had been a world still at the mercy of bacterial infection, with hospital wards then filled with women dying of the 'childbed fever'. She was there to watch the most extraordinary transformation as antibiotics were widely introduced, and countless lives were saved. In perhaps the greatest irony, I am now working at the frontier of a new epidemic, which may have its origins in this victory over the bacterial world. But back as I listened to these stories, the allergy epidemic was only beginning to show and was still not recognised by most.

I also learned that it was there in medical school that Monica met my grandfather, Stanley. He fell in love with her immediately. Until he met Monica, Stanley had not planned to leave England. But her passion was contagious and he soon went to China to learn the language while she finished her medical training. A year later, Monica sailed to Hong Kong to be reunited with her fiancé, only days before war broke out in North China. The Japanese invasion left Stanley stranded in the heart of the war zone. I loved hearing how the newspapers told of Stanley's perilous 1300 mile journey down the Chinese coast in small Chinese junks and fishing boats, slipping past Japanese warships at Shanghai in the dead of night, to claim his bride. It was even more incredible to hear how, together, they braved the typhoons and returned to the war zone of North China where Monica set to work as a doctor and Stanley became the youngest medical superintendent of the Qilu Hospital. For the next three years they provided much needed medical care to the war-ravaged Chinese, always under the watchful eyes of the Japanese soldiers. This was where my father, David, was born. He was only eighteen months old when hostilities escalated and they had to join the British evacuation or face life in a concentration camp. Stanley chose to stay behind to keep the hospital running as long as he could, while Monica and David joined the other refugees on a very long, crowded and uncertain ocean journey south. They arrived safely in Australia before their ship was sunk in Darwin harbour by the Japanese. After many months of uncertainty, Stanley finally escaped on one of the last boats out. Leaving their home in China, they made a new life in Australia. Stanley went on to become one of the longest serving Vice Chancellors of the University of Western Australia (UWA), where I now work. From humble beginnings, Sir Stanley and Lady Prescott found themselves at Royal garden parties, and when the queen visited Australia, they were invited to dine with her on the *Britannia*. But they never lost their humility or their sense of what was important.

Through this, I could see how a passion for helping people find love, health and spiritual sustenance molded my family and brought us to Australia. Monica had succeeded in igniting my passion and a strong commitment to study medicine. I just had to hope for good enough exam results, and wished I had thought of this *before* I sat my exams. My conviction further deepened when Monica told me that it was Stanley who founded the first Medical School in Western Australia.

I think Monica was as nervous as I during the wait for my exam results. We were dining in a hotel in London when my father called me from Australia with the news. He could hardly speak and started by telling me that the numbers were so low that he had to call the authorities to see if there was some mistake. I was already feeling sick as he explained that he had been looking at my state ranking and not my aggregate score, which was so large that he also could hardly believe it. Neither could I. Although I had always done well in school, I had no way of knowing how I might do in the state ranking. Still in happy shock, I returned to the dining table to tell my good news. I had never seen Monica look so proud and that was the best moment. So, with the sense of anticipation, wonder and adventure I share with my ancestors, I set off on my own path. A door of the universe had opened to me and I felt my own calling to go through. How could I not?

• • •

I clearly needed to use my head to study medicine, but my philosophy has always been to follow my heart first and foremost, to do what felt right and what made me happiest. One of Stanley's final duties as the Chairman of Royal Perth Hospital was to recruit a new and brilliant Professor of Medicine, Professor Lawrie Beilin, who was also to play a critical role in my career. As a fourth year medical student in 1985, I somehow found myself in Prof. Beilin's office, metres from where Stanley had presided over the opening of the medical school. I can't really remember how I came to be sitting alone before his desk without my fellow students. I think he was reflecting fondly of how he appreciated my grandfather's belief in him. Perhaps he wanted to repay the favour in some way. In any case, he gave me an opportunity for which I will be forever grateful. I took it, without question. In my heart I knew it was the right thing to do. My fellow students did not understand the attraction of taking a year off from my medical training to undertake a year of research, and write an honours thesis. Incomprehensible. Studying medicine took long enough as it was. But it was my first taste of academic life, and I don't regret it for a moment. Monica, as ever, was pleased and excited by my decision. Many years later in 1999, when I was appointed as a tenured academic at UWA, one of my first and most fruitful collaborations was with Lawrie Beilin's group. Although we worked in very different fields by then, that very diversity paved the way for some quite novel research.

I worked very hard when I returned to the ranks of medical school, but I tried to not take life too seriously and do what I could to retain perspective. Two weeks before my final medical exams, when my classmates were all madly cramming in a climate of growing stress and paranoia, I decided to follow a different tack. We had a series of written and oral exams. Standing alone in front of examiners, who had the power to throw almost anything at us, was the moment of intimidation that we had all been dreading for six years. We could not even imagine life after that moment. I knew I had done the work. What I really needed now was perspective, clarity and a sense of humour. The best way to achieve all of these was immediately obvious. I needed to travel. Travel to the other side of an unknown universe. So off I went with Douglas Adams and his *Hitchhikers Guide*. Ten days before my exams I embarked on this grand journey reading every book in the *Hitchhikers Guide,* before returning to Earth just in time to meet my examiners. Fresh. Inspired. Ready for anything. It certainly gave me another perspective. And I never expected to have so much fun. I had a great time and did well. And I am sure that a universal perspective mixed with humble confidence helped.

The intern year was another challenge. I picked up my first pager with all the other nervous interns and ran to hide in the toilets as I waited for it to go off for the first time. It did not take long. A few major traumas and cardiac arrests later and soon I was in the full swing of things. It was also not long before my classmates started to choose specialty-training programs. But after a full year of internal medicine I still had not found my calling. It was overwhelming, exhausting and I was just too tired and disillusioned to feel inspired. Being assaulted by intoxicated and uncooperative patients in the Emergency Department did not help. I started to wonder if I might be on the right path after all. This might have contributed to my decision to take a dramatic detour in my second year. Struggling for direction and involved with a boy about to go overseas, I considered dropping out for a year, maybe more, hoping that things would clarify. I just knew I didn't want to stay where I was. In what most of my friends and family believed was a misguided choice; I decided to follow the boy. It was an ill-fated relationship and a detour that could have turned into a cul-de-sac. But it didn't. As life often does, the painful and seemingly pointless detour actually led me far more quickly to purpose and direction. Within a few months I found myself stranded, literally, on an island in the middle of the Pacific. No boy. No money. No idea. To make ends meet I worked for the Fiji School of Medicine doing some basic research. This achieved important two things. It reinforced my love of research. And it was there that I met the man who inspired my passion to study paediatics, Professor Ian Lewis, a retired Australian paediatrician heading the Fiji medical school. Seeing my interest and clear attraction to paediatrics, he mapped it all out clearly for me. Go back to Perth. Enter into paediatric residency for three years of basic training. Sit my paediatric exams. Pass the first time, although that is hard to do. Enter three more years of advanced training. Oh, and do a PhD at the same time. Sure. I nodded. Like hell! After seven years of medical school this did not sound like much fun.

But paediatrics 'felt' like a good idea, so why not? I decided to do that for a while to see what might happen. Unfortunately I discovered paediatrics was so popular that when I initially applied all the jobs were taken, with no prospects for at least a year. So I actually had to trudge back to Royal Perth Hospital and work in the Emergency Department again. Not my favorite place. But now my intensions were set and I was happy. As chance would have it, I was almost immediately and unexpectedly seconded to the Emergency Department at the Children's hospital. I literally came in the back door, and I never left. So I like to think of it as destiny that, within six months of setting my intentions in Fiji, I found myself back in Perth studying paediatrics. And six years later I took great joy in writing to Ian Lewis to let him know that everything had unfolded *exactly* as he planned, with the PhD thrown in for good measure. His soothsaying had not extended to what my chosen specialty should be, so I had to figure that out for myself.

. . .

Immunology and Allergy was one of the most intimidating and the most hated specialties when we were in medical school. A little later you will see why. After graduation it did not get any more popular in attracting specialty trainees. No one in my cohort was drawn to specialise in this field. But I like a challenge. At that stage there were many new and confusing discoveries about the immune system, and its role in so many diseases and conditions was starting to become more recognised. The current crisis of food allergy was still unheard of, but asthma was becoming more common, and the first speculations that this might be related to the decline in bacterial infectious diseases were only just starting to emerge. Still, very little was known about the developing immune system in early life, when bacterial exposure seemed most critical for maturation of immune function. And around the time I was starting my advanced training, I had the chance to research this topic and answer this important question. By working in the allergy clinics and undertaking a PhD at the same time, I had the perfect opportunity to study exactly how the immune system develops and how this goes wrong in allergic children. I got that 'feeling' again. It was the right thing to do.

And it was. Under the inspiring tutelage of Professor Patrick Holt, I undertook important work that was soon published in the *Lancet* and which had great impact on our understanding of the early immune system and how we think about allergic disease. The enormous interest in my work launched my international career. So although I am still not exactly sure what I want to be when I grow up, this seems to be a good start.

It is hard not to be amazed when I reflect on just how much

medicine has changed since my grandmother Monica was in medical school fifty years before me. From a world plagued with infectious diseases, to a much cleaner world now plagued with allergy and many other immune diseases. My specialty did not even exist in Monica's day. Now looking at the new generation of medical students in front of me, I can't help but wonder what lies in store for them.

3

In the classroom: some basics of allergy

Time to get down to business and learn more about allergic disease. I like to start by reminding the medical students just how common and serious allergies can be, and how fast this problem has been increasing. When I started medical school in the early 1980s, allergy was hardly mentioned at all. There was some teaching on asthma but without much focus on the underlying inflammation or the links with the immune system. Even long after I graduated, many respiratory specialists remained doubtful about the relevance of allergy. As medical students we did learn about skin inflammation in eczema, but our dermatology teachers were equally skeptical about any link with allergy. And I did not even hear about food allergy until some years after I graduated. At that stage, the field of Allergy was a very, very poor cousin to the fairly new field of Immunology, which was more focussed on immune deficiencies. There were very few advocates for Allergy and only a few took it seriously. That has certainly changed. Now most community doctors are seeing evidence of the allergy epidemic on a daily basis, and the medical curriculum has caught up with this change in disease profile.

Before the students learn about disease they need a basic understanding of the normal immune system and a general grounding in what causes the allergic response. These students have already done some of the basics in their earlier training, so we begin by reviewing the following basic points about allergy and what happens during an allergic reaction.

WHAT IS ALLERGY?

We remind the students that in the most basic terms, allergy occurs when there is a seemingly pointless immune response to completely harmless factors in the environment.

One of the main functions of the immune system is to protect our bodies from infections and other possible dangers in the environment. Allergic individuals direct this immune attack at things that do not present any real threat, such as proteins in foods and pollens. In this case the attacker is the only one that suffers in this misdirected assault. This self-damaging allergic response causes inflammation, which leads to the signs and symptoms of allergic disease. These symptoms depend on where in the body the reaction occurs.

As allergic reactions are directed to the external environment, it makes sense that the areas of the body affected are those that are in most immediate contact with the environment: the skin, the airways and the gut. Reactions that occur mainly in the skin lead to hives or to eczema, a form of dermatitis. Reactions to inhaled environmental particles can be seen in the nose as rhinitis and in the lower airways of the lungs as asthma. While reactions to ingested foods are seen in the gut, the effects are often more extensive with more generalised symptoms (see Chapter 11) which can even be life threatening. Severe and generalised reactions can also occur when allergens directly penetrate tissues or the blood stream, as we commonly see with insect sting allergies.

WHAT ARE ALLERGENS?

'Allergen' is the name we give to virtually *anything* that triggers an allergic response. So potentially *anything* in the environment can be an allergen. In other words, allergens are the 'target' that the immune system illogically singles out. However, there do appear to be certain things that are more 'allergenic' than others, making them more likely targets of the immune system. This is the reason that certain allergies are more common. For example, the most common food proteins to cause reactions are found in eggs, cow's milk, peanut, soy, tree nuts and seafood, and the inhaled proteins most likely to induce reactions are found in dust mites, animal dander and pollens. The 'top ten' allergens vary according to geographical region, depending on which allergens are most prevalent in that environment. Allergens are usually proteins, although there are a few rare exceptions, and the pattern of response is generally similar regardless of the trigger.

The allergic response is very selective. An allergic person will encounter countless different proteins over their lifetime, and they will produce perfectly normal responses to virtually all of these potential allergens. They only mount an allergic immune response to a select few. Even the most allergic people only make allergic antibodies to a tiny fraction of the possible allergens that they encounter in the environment.

There are a number of possible reasons that some substances are more allergenic. Some allergenic proteins have been shown to have chemical or enzymic properties that might make them more irritating. This seems to fool the immune system into thinking that the allergen poses a threat. Some of these allergens, such as dust mite proteins, also have structural elements similar to bacterial products, which normally induce an immune response. One theory is that when our immune system is too busy fighting real infection, as it was in centuries gone by, it is less likely to be distracted by any of these allergen protein imposters. But this does not fully explain exactly why the allergens evoke allergic antibodies, and not typical defensive antibodies.

ALLERGENS ARE NOT TO BLAME

One thing we must remember is that allergens are just the 'target' of the immune response; they themselves do not appear to cause the underlying allergy. Allergens can certainly not explain the epidemic rise in allergy, which is more likely to be due to other environmental forces effectively 'loading the gun' by altering the immune system such that allergic responses are more likely. We should be looking for what is loading the gun rather than at the target.

Allergenic foods like milk and eggs have been part of our diets for thousands of years, but allergies to these have only appeared very recently. Although it might seem obvious now that allergens could not possibly be responsible for the general rise in allergy and other immune diseases, this has been a common and longstanding misconception. In fact, it has only been quite recently, in 2008, that experts around the world stopped recommending 'allergen avoidance' in early life to prevent the development of allergic disease.[1] After nearly twenty years of failed attempts to avert the allergy epidemic by avoiding the most allergenic foods and inhaled allergens, it is not surprising that this change in approach has been quite confusing for the community. But we must remember that these guidelines were based on the best evidence available at the time (see Chapter 9).[2] As we learn more, our perspective changes. It has taken time and research to revise these practices. Importantly, as we gain more knowledge, we need to prepare for further possible changes. But at least we have the insight to know we are nowhere near the end of this story yet.

WHAT HAPPENS DURING AN ALLERGIC REACTION?

There are several different kinds of reactions to allergens. In broad terms, allergic reactions are mediated by antibodies or cells that have been conditioned to attack allergens. We will come back later to how these responses get conditioned, but once these antibodies and cells are present in significant numbers, any encounter with an allergen will typically trigger a reaction.

The most common kind of reaction is the sudden (acute) reaction, which is mediated by allergic antibodies. These antibodies are from the immunoglobulin E (IgE) group of antibodies, which induce sudden swelling, rashes and itching along with other symptoms depending on where the reaction occurs. Each antibody can only recognise a particular allergen. Unless they come across that allergen, absolutely nothing happens. Everyone has some IgE to various things, but whereas non-allergic individuals only have low levels, allergic individuals have much higher levels of IgE that are directed to the particular allergen(s) they are allergic to. These antibodies circulate in the blood and are found in tissue where they bind to histamine containing cells called 'mast' cells (Figure 1).

When we do allergy tests, we are looking for the presence or levels of IgE antibodies to specific allergens (see Chapter 10). IgE antibodies were not discovered until the 1960s and are quite different to the IgG antibodies which fight bacterial infections and which do not cause histamine release.

The allergic response only occurs when an allergen binds to the IgE on the cell surface and sets off a rapid 'chain reaction'. Even tiny amounts of allergen can trigger this response.

For example, the child with peanut allergy will have a large number of IgE molecules in their blood (Figure 1a) and on their mast cell surfaces (Figure 1b) and a high proportion of these will be directed to peanut. Nothing happens until this child comes into contact with peanuts. When the peanut allergens bind the many peanut-specific IgE receptors in the mast cell surface, these IgE molecules become interlinked into a matrix, which induces the cell to spill histamine and other chemical mediators into the tissues (Figure 1c). Other cells called eosinophils also play a major role in the acute allergic response pouring more inflammatory chemicals into the tissues.

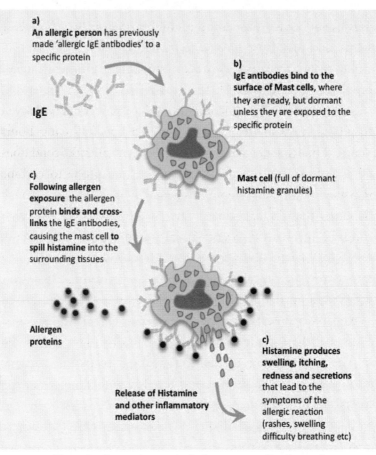

a)
An allergic person has previously made 'allergic IgE antibodies' to a specific protein

IgE

b)
IgE antibodies bind to the surface of Mast cells, where they are ready, but dormant unless they are exposed to the specific protein

c)
Following allergen exposure the allergen protein **binds and cross-links** the IgE antibodies, causing the mast cell **to spill histamine** into the surrounding tissues

Mast cell (full of dormant histamine granules)

Allergen proteins

Release of Histamine and other inflammatory mediators

c)
Histamine produces swelling, itching, redness and secretions that lead to the symptoms of the allergic reaction (rashes, swelling difficulty breathing etc)

Figure 1   Events that occur during an acute allergic attack

It is the histamine and related mediators such as leukotrienes that cause all the signs and symptoms of the allergic reaction such as itching, redness and swelling (Figure 1d). As discussed later, the effects can range from unpleasant (such as itching or vomiting) to life threatening (if it occurs in the throat and blocks breathing). Once a reaction has occurred, the symptoms usually settle spontaneously, although serious reactions should be terminated quickly with treatment.

It is very reasonable to question why these IgE antibodies evolved in the first place, if they cause so many problems. This family of antibodies is actually a normal part of our body's defense systems, and they have evolved to particularly attack parasites. In societies that encounter very few parasites, these antibodies appear more likely to be misdirected to attack allergens (see Chapter 8).

Sometimes the IgE reaction also induces a secondary delayed 'late-phase' reaction that can evolve over the following hours or days. This is more common in persistent allergic conditions such as asthma and eczema, where tissues are prone to chronic (long-standing) inflammation. It is generally mediated by immune cells rather than by antibodies. The chemical mediators released during the IgE reaction recruit more immune cells to the site of the reaction where they can perpetuate the inflammation. The IgE response is the most common kind of allergic reaction, but there are others. These are much less common and are driven by cellular responses which do not involve IgE at all. The best examples of these kinds of cell-mediated reactions are seen in the gut. They generally occur hours after ingesting the food trigger and are still not fully understood. As IgE is not involved, the patients do not experience histamine-related symptoms. Instead they have diarrhoea, vomiting and related symptoms. This can be harder to diagnose because the IgE allergy test is usually negative (see Chapter 11).

• • •

All of the students have had some lectures on these basics earlier in their courses, so once we have completed the review, we get down to business and focus on allergy case studies. The students take turns to present cases of real patients with common allergies that they have just seen in the clinics. After telling the patients' stories, students discuss the research evidence that applies to each case. Some of these cases are outlined later in Chapters 11–15.

They do the work. They quiz each other. My role at this

point is to make sure that the discussions are dynamic and the facts are correct. I often supervise role-playing where one student will act as a doctor giving advice or explaining how to use an adrenaline auto-injector to another student pretending to be a patient or a parent. We create real-life scenarios that they are likely to encounter in general practice.

The idea of this kind of learning is that the students are actively engaged rather than passively dozing in a lecture. Their practical exams at the end of the year run in a very similar role-play scenario format. As always, the students are more focussed on passing exams than on their future practice, but at least we make sure that the skills they learn are directly relevant for both.

Each group of students is different, which keeps it interesting for me too. The underlying issues might be the same, but there are always so many new patients to discuss. Many changes have happened in the field over the last ten–fifteen years that I have been teaching, and this form of dynamic, evidence-based learning ensures the students are keeping up to date with the latest approaches.

I love it most when I see the students discover controversies and uncertainties. And there are still plenty. Although it is unsettling at first, it is critical for students to realise that we don't have all the answers. Above all, they must learn that ongoing research is essential to understand both the big picture of the allergy crisis as well as all of the specific questions that it raises.

When they come to the edge of the unknown, their interest is most stimulated. They realise that what they are learning now is only the beginning of a story that will continue to evolve over their lifetime. With any luck, we always hope to find a few who choose to join our ranks in the adventure of that discovery.

4

On the world stage: a global perspective

Stepping out of the classroom I have to change gear again. Although mildly exhausted, I always find my time with the students uplifting. Their questions give perspective and meaning to all the other work that we do. But now I have to gather my thoughts for a lecture I will be giving in London in two days. I will be on a plane again all day tomorrow and I have not even packed yet. There are always last minute changes to my PowerPoint presentation, and I am glad we no longer have to prepare projector slides by hand weeks ahead. With the pace of life today, I don't think many of us would cope with that now.

Before I rush home to get ready, I check in with my research team, grateful to hear that everything seems to be okay. The PhD students, the research assistants, and the research nurses are all busy. My senior research scientists give me a brief up-date and I am out the door. Back to Europe for the second time this month.

I am very fortunate to be part of the international community of experts all working to understand the allergy epidemic. Because the work of my research team is internationally recognised, I am frequently invited to meetings all around the world to present our findings, discuss new issues and to form new collaborations. I also feel very privileged to be working as a member of the World Allergy Organization (WAO). The mission of the WAO is to be a global resource and advocate in the field of allergy, asthma and clinical immunology, and to advance excellence in clinical care through education, research and training. As a worldwide alliance, the Organization presently embraces more than eighty regional and national allergy, asthma and clinical immunology societies and affiliated organisations. In response to the growing concern about the increasing global burden of allergic diseases, a major focus of the organisation is to create global awareness of allergy and asthma as a major public health problem, In 2011, the WAO presented the first ever global *White Book on Allergy* which is now publicly available at <www.worldallergy.org> as a resource for health care workers, governments and policy makers around the globe.

The chance to meet with colleagues from other regions is a critical part of our work. This provides fertile ground for new ideas and new angles for tackling the issues. Some of the largest international meetings on allergy are held each year in Europe and North America, with scores of invited lecturers like me, and often more than 5,000 delegates from around the world. It is both humbling and a privilege to stand before such large audiences of my peers.

I have to do a lot of public speaking now. Friends often ask, faced with such a large audience, what do you do? Visualise them all in their underwear? Well no. Not me. I delve into the place that I found before my exams, the place that I can feel perspective, energy, fun and levity, and truly feel the power of the present moment. Ironically, most of our lives we are not 'present' but preoccupied with the past or worrying about the future. The moments before stepping onto a stage can give the most focus, the most intense and powerful experience of being completely 'in the present'. Energy and adrenalin are surging, but I feel perfectly still. Perfectly calm as everything else melts away. A rare and precious feeling to capture in our otherwise busy and distracted lives.

There are many other speakers at these meetings and so many diverse areas of research; we all have much to learn from each other. Some researchers focus on the genetics of allergic disease, some on the environmental causes. Others focus their research on better clinical treatment or prevention of disease. Yet others examine the many different aspects of the underlying immune system which might cause allergy and provide targets for new treatments. This provides a true melting pot, where new ideas are born.

As I board the plane, I am still inspired by my patients' questions to make this information publicly accessible, and it is on the flight that I start to commit some of these words to the page. With the knowledge that the allergy story is an 'international work in progress' that will evolve much further in the years to come, I still feel that we have to start somewhere. We should not wait until we think we have all the answers; that might be a long time coming.

A GLOBAL CRISIS: ALLERGY IS PART OF A MUCH BIGGER PROBLEM

When we all come together at these large international meetings it is hard to miss the global scale of the allergy epidemic. Yet we now see that it is only one part of a much, much larger problem. We are now living in an era of more immune disease in general. Over the last fifty years there has been a massive rise in a whole range of immune conditions including allergic diseases, inflammatory bowel diseases, multiple sclerosis, rheumatoid arthritis, thyroid disease and insulin dependent diabetes, to name but a few.

It has taken decades for us to recognise the consequences of progressive industrialisation on the health of our planet. And now we are seeing the effects on our own health. While many body systems are sensitive to environmental change, the impact on the immune system has been dramatic. The enormous rise in immune diseases over a relatively short period is the clearest evidence of this.

While these many immune diseases affect different body organs and have quite different symptoms, they all have one common thread: they are due to abnormal 'rogue' immune cells that damage these various organs and tissues (see Chapter 5). This can only happen because these renegade cells are allowed to escape normal immune control in the first place.

The immune system is designed to recognise and eradicate cells which are 'out of control' and potentially harmful. But if these escape surveillance, they multiply, making countless identical 'clones' of themselves to cause disease. In each of these diseases, the renegade clones selectively attack a particular target. The nature of that target determines the kind of disease we see (figure 2).[1] It might seem like the clones are winning this battle, but we are not defeated.

The fact that so many of these immune diseases have increased over the same period is a major clue that environmental changes are affecting the underlying 'master control' of immune function. In other words, the regulatory surveillance divisions of the

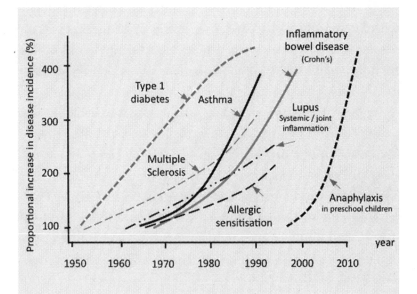

Figure 2 Dramatic rise in many immune diseases – an epidemic of allergy and autoimmune disease

immune system appear less effective, so rogue clones are more likely to escape control.

A breakdown of immune surveillance, however subtle, may have even broader implications than we first suspected: these are also the very same systems that we depend on to recognise and kill off cancerous clones before they can develop into malignant cancers. The immune system is even implicated in conditions such as heart disease, obesity, and high blood pressure, which are now known to be associated with increased inflammation. It may be no coincidence that all of these other conditions have been on the rise during the very same period. In fact, there is now grow-ing speculation that these apparently diverse conditions may all be interlinked in ways that we are only just beginning to understand.[2]

We hope that the mysteries of each of these individual conditions may be revealed by a better understanding of their interrelationships.

We are only just beginning to recognise the significance of these interconnections, and this is the reason that there is now intense scientific interest in the 'regulatory' immune cells and what influences these (Chapter 5).

The immune system reaches into virtually every organ and every structure. It is essential for normal health and function. If we hope to solve this modern health crisis, we must have a better understanding of the environmental factors that are driving this growing tendency for inflammation (see Prime Suspects in Chapter 8), as well as how the underlying immune processes are affected. Finding the common threads between the rise in allergies and these other conditions may hold vital clues.

THE SCALE OF THE ALLERGY EPIDEMIC
The rise in allergic disease first began in the more industrially developed countries of Australasia, Western Europe and North

America. However, the same patterns are becoming equally apparent in virtually all regions of the world undergoing industrial development and westernisation.[3] Burgeoning rates of allergic disease in populous developing countries in Asia, Africa and South America[4] highlight that this is fast becoming a global health issue of major importance.

This is another clear indicator of the power of environmental change to affect immune function regardless of genetic background. As the highly populated countries of Asia are becoming affected, the numbers of people involved are likely to escalate beyond anything we anticipated. This is now truly a global epidemic. Recent studies show that allergies are rising even in populations such as the indigenous islanders of Papua New Guinea, who were previously unaffected.[5]

The rates and patterns of allergy still vary greatly between regions and with age. In highly westernised countries like Australia around 40 per cent of the population is estimated to have allergic antibodies to common harmless environmental proteins ('allergens')[6] from dust mites, pets, pollens and foods. Not all of these people will develop actual allergic disease, but a high proportion will. Asthma is still one of the most common allergic diseases, particularly in children, with as many as 20–25 per cent of children affected by asthma symptoms (such as wheezing) in some studies. 'Hay-fever' (allergic rhinitis) affects an even higher proportion of the population, although this tends to begin later in childhood and adulthood, affecting more than 40 per cent of some populations at some stage in their lives.[7] While the rates of asthma appear to have reached a peak in most developed countries,[8] other allergic diseases such as food allergy and eczema (dermatitis) are clearly still rising.[9] These conditions occur most commonly in young infants. Studies indicate that at least 15 per cent of infants this age have eczema and at least 6 per cent have food allergy;[10] but that number is probably much higher.[11] It can take many years to gather data on the rate of allergy, so even the most recent data can already be out of date.[12] With that in mind, it is very likely that these figures significantly underestimate the allergy rates in many areas.

SOCIAL AND ECONOMIC COSTS: PREVENTION IS BETTER THAN CURE

With these trends it is easy to imagine the enormous impact on societies. Although the individuals with allergies face the most immediate burden of disease, with the associated stresses, social and financial costs, the impact of the allergy epidemic is quickly flowing on to the whole community.

The current economic costs are unparalleled. In most developed countries, *billions* of dollars are spent each year treating allergic diseases, and this figure is rising. In the United States these costs doubled between 2000 and 2005, reaching more than $11 billion per year.[13] Even in much smaller countries like Australia, where allergy rates are arguably the highest in the world, the costs are incredible. A 2007 report outlined how the financial cost of allergies in Australia was $7.8 billion, with lost productivity and health system expenditure the major contributing factors.[14] This number blew out further to $21.5 billion per year when the impact of reduced quality of life (the 'burden of disease') was also included. This is approximately double the estimated figures for other common conditions such as arthritis ($11.7 billion for 2007 in Australia).[15]

These figures are staggering, and remind us that 'prevention is better than cure'. While this increased expenditure on treatment is essential to respond to the problem and treat those who are already affected by disease, we need to look beyond that. We spend very little on disease prevention. We also spend relatively little on finding real cures. And in the absence of cures, most current health expenditure goes towards symptom relief. This applies to almost all areas of health.

In the longer term, it is more important for our governments to invest in prevention strategies that might arrest or reverse this epidemic. Pouring money into band-aid treatment will not achieve this. Getting this balance right is an age-old dilemma, and in short-term economic policies prevention inevitably loses out.

We all hope that we will turn the page, and that the twenty-first century will herald a new era in health where the focus is on promoting health through disease prevention. This makes perfect sense at both the economic level and the personal level; it depends on long-term investment and a long-range vision. Just as it has taken a critical mass of collective 'believers' for governments to start addressing the crisis in our natural environment, the same is true of human health. It will take time, but the seeds are there. We all have a role to play.

Food allergy: a worrying 'second wave' to the allergy epidemic

This brings us to another great puzzle. The allergy epidemic began with the rise in respiratory diseases such as asthma and rhinitis that are associated with allergies to inhaled allergens (from mites, pollens, pets). This began over fifty years ago and was in full swing in developed countries by the 1980s. At that stage, there was some evidence of food allergy and eczema but the rates were much lower than they are today. The rise in allergies associated with ingested (food) allergens has been much more recent.

So why has there been a twenty year lag between the 'inhalant' and the 'food' allergy epidemics?[16]

There is virtually no doubt that the increase in food allergy is real. Although people are certainly more aware of food allergy, and more likely to go to the doctor, this cannot explain the scale of the increasing rates of diagnosis, particularly in young infants. Food allergy reactions can be severe and dramatic; not the kind of thing that is easily overlooked by the unaware.

34

As with the asthma epidemic, countries like Australia, the United Kingdom and the United States are again leading the way in the food allergy epidemic.[17] But other regions are now showing the same trends. Because of the rapid changes and the time it takes to collect new data, it is difficult to get accurate current data on food allergy rates. Recent preliminary data from a survey of community health clinics in Victoria (Australia) shows that more than 20 per cent of one year olds have positive allergy tests to common foods such as egg, milk and peanuts.[18] At least half of these had an allergic reaction, such as swelling, rash or vomiting when they were given a supervised test feed (food challenge). This is consistent with the growing numbers of parents reporting food reactions, and the four-fold increase in emergency department visits with life-threatening anaphylactic reactions to foods over a decade.[19] All of these observations strongly suggest that food allergy is much more common than ever before and that it is still on the rise.

As part of this phenomenon we also see the first signs of allergy at much earlier ages with food allergies and eczema often first appearing in the first weeks and months of life.

At this stage we cannot explain the secondary rise in food allergy and why this has been delayed. One thing is clear, the environmental pressures that are causing this rise in infant allergy must be acting very early in life, even before birth (see Chapter 6). And in the future, this period of life may indeed provide the best window of opportunity for preventing allergic disease and reversing the allergy epidemic.

LIGHT AT THE END OF THE TUNNEL

My purpose in highlighting the problems we face is not to spread doom and gloom. Quite the opposite. Part of solving a problem is recognising and understanding it. We have only recently begun to see the scale of this problem and there are now literally thousands of researchers working to understand this better. Both government and community awareness around the globe has helped channel research funds into solving these problems, and it is important that this continues. New perspectives will bring new approaches. We are already starting to see this.

Although immune disease is one of the prices we pay for modern living, we have every reason to hope that there will be ways of overcoming this. The answers are likely to be right in front of us; we just have to understand them. The very fact that environmental change has caused an increase in disease tells us that there is 'plasticity' in the immune system, and that immune development can be molded by the environment. We can hope to harness that same plasticity and *use the environment* to prevent disease before it develops or to reprogram errant responses once they have developed. To do that we need to better understand how the environment alters the expression of our genes.

These are the many issues that we discuss and debate at our international meetings. But, while we devote considerable time to these large-scale visions, this is balanced in equal measure by detailed discussions exploring the microscopic events in the immune system which lead to allergic disease. Without a good understanding of the immune system, we cannot hope to prevent immune diseases.

5

Down the rabbit hole: into the immune system

Here we go, like Alice, down the rabbit hole into the amazing parallel universe of the immune system. There we will meet weird and wonderful characters, of many shapes and sizes. We will find large armies as well as lone sentinels. There will be assassins and noble warriors. Some will be naïve, and others well trained. Most will be loyal defenders of their kingdom, but we will surely discover mutinous renegades among them. This is a vast world we knew nothing of when Alice began her own adventures in Wonderland in 1865. And we still have much left to explore.

THE QUICK 'POTTED' VERSION FOR THOSE WHO DON'T WANT TO DO THE FULL TOUR OF THE IMMUNE SYSTEM

Before we go any further, this tour of the immune system will divide into two groups. For those who are game and want to stay with me on the main tour, we will take an excursion to see the major highlights of the immune system and meet some of the strange creatures that inhabit this space. But a small warning; the first time you enter this world you don't have to venture far before getting mind meltdown. So, for those who want to only take a quick look through the window, this is my way of giving you full permission to take a break and avoid any unpleasant brain explosions in the middle of an immunology tour.

For those who prefer the break but don't want to miss anything important, here are the summary highlights, which will also serve as a beginner's guide for those of you who do want to come with me a little further into this wondrous world of the immune system.

The basics of the immune system

1. We are all born with some 'basic' immunity

There are a number of cells that are 'hard wired' to defend against threats. Even newborn babies have these 'innate' immune cells that provide some basic inherent protection without any need for conditioning or pre-programming. These cells start the process, but need to call for help from more efficient and more specialised defense teams. But specialised defenses are naïve and immature at birth, and have to be trained by the innate cells before they can make more efficient responses. Every time the innate cells see something new, they digest it into small pieces (called antigens) and present these pieces to the immature specialised defense cells to teach them about the environment and to program them to make more efficient responses when they encounter the antigen again in the future. These innate 'antigen presenting cells' also secrete signals (called cytokines) that influence the pattern of response.

2. The main cells in specialised defense are the B cells and the T cells

B cells make antibodies that are directed at neutralising a specific protein (antigen). Some T cells can kill or try to destroy the antigen they have been trained to recognise, others help B cells make antibodies and produce cytokine signals to tell B cells what kind of antibodies to make (i.e. whether to make allergic antibodies or normal defense antibodies).

3. Turning off an immune response is just as important

Once a threat has passed, the immune reaction must be switched off quickly, or we would soon die from uncontrolled inflammation. There are a number of mechanisms that do this including 'regulatory cells' and 'regulatory cytokines' which have inhibitory effects on other immune cells.

What seems to go wrong with this system in allergy?

At some point after innate cells have presented antigen to the T cells, the T cells 'decide' to produce Type 2 allergic cytokines instead of normal Type 1 defense responses. It is not clear if this fault lies with the messages received from innate cells during the T cell programming, or if this defect is intrinsic to T cells, or both. The Type 2 cytokines then induce the B cells to make allergic IgE antibodies which are responsible for all of the signs and symptoms of allergy. Inadequate inhibitory signals from regulatory cells may also play a role in allowing an allergic response to become more established. Bacterial exposure stimulates innate cells and promotes the Type 1 responses, which are important for microbial defense, and which also inhibit Type 2 allergic responses. Bacteria also promote activation of regulatory cells. This is why it has been proposed that cleaner environments could be promoting allergic disease by sending inadequate signals to the Type 1 and regulatory cells, allowing the Type 2 responses to expand unchecked.

So follow me now, those who want to know more about the lives of these characters and how and why they do what they do. For the others, we will see you on the other side, at Chapter 6.

THE MAIN TOUR OF THE IMMUNE SYSTEM STARTS HERE!

As I am sure you already suspect, there is nothing simple about the immune system. It is incredibly complex. We immunologists have not helped by making our descriptive models so ridiculously complicated. There are so many aspects to it, and amazingly, we are discovering new pathways and new relationships every year. It is not surprising that recent generations of medical students have found this so intimidating. But rather than be overwhelmed, we should marvel at the intricacies of this extraordinary system and what it can achieve.

There are vast networks of cells, all with different functions, constantly interacting at lightning speed. It is like a high-speed internet. Everything is interconnected, constantly changing and evolving in response to every interaction with the environment. The static models and labels that we use to understand and describe this web of activity are woefully inadequate in describing what happens in real-time. By their very nature, scientific models tend to be more black and white than reality. Models are very useful, but we must be aware of their limitations. Nothing is cut and dried when it comes to the immune system. So keep that in mind as we start to explore some of the basics of the immune response through the eyes of current science. As we start to learn more, we accept that these models are likely to change. In the last twenty years we have already seen some major shifts in these models. The only way to stay sane while studying immunology is to surrender and accept the fact that we can never understand it all. The more we discover, the more we realise there is yet more beyond our grasp. And while this system must logically be finite, there is no sign that we are approaching the end.

In any situation, the immune system must tread a very narrow path between adequate, defensive responses and inappropriate (pathological) immune responses as in allergic disease and self-destructive autoimmune responses. It must produce enough inflammation to eradicate infections, but make sure that this is contained, self-limiting and not directed at the wrong targets. Considering the vast number of foreign and 'self' proteins (i.e. the many proteins that belong to the body) that the immune system encounters every minute of every day, it is miraculous that it does not make more errors.

DEVELOPING IMMUNE MEMORIES

Although cells in the first line of defense are 'hard wired' to react to danger signals, these are not as efficient as the specialised second-line cells which actually have to go through a training program of sorts in order to 'learn' about the specific environment. These secondary, professional hit cells are conditioned after they first see a foreign protein, so they can respond more quickly and more effectively if they see it again. Some also produce showers of antibodies to help in this very efficiently targeted attack. This ability to develop immune 'memory' is what allows us to adapt and protect ourselves in diverse environments. Our individual patterns of immune memory reflect all of the environmental proteins that we have seen, including infections, vaccines and allergens.

It is these memory cells that also mount allergic responses. This can really only occur if they have seen the allergen or something very similar to it before. Non-allergic people also have immune 'memory' of the allergens that their system has encountered, but the key difference in allergic individuals is not in *whether* they have memory, but *how* their memory cells respond.

In essence, allergic responses are due to abnormal memory responses that promote IgE production. Scientists have arbitrarily labeled these as 'Type 2' memory responses, to distinguish them from the 'Type 1' non-allergic memory responses.

THE MAIN PLAYERS IN PROGRAMMING IMMUNE MEMORY

We are born with 'inbuilt' defense cells that respond rapidly to an immediate threat. They don't need to have memory of foreign proteins (antigens) to react to them. These front-line cells are sometimes called 'innate' immune cells. They detect danger signals such as tissue damage. The mast cells of the allergic reaction (Chapter 3) are part of this innate defense system.

Antigen Presenting Cells (APC): a first line of 'innate' defense
There are many other cells with innate defense capacity, but the one that is most relevant here is the 'antigen presenting cell' (APC). These are fascinating to look at. Some have many long projections, like arms, that make them look like octopuses (Figure 3). These particular APC (called dendritic cells or 'DC' because of their shape), roam around in our tissues literally looking for any signs of trouble. This surveillance team sticks their long arms up as probes through the mucous membranes in the gut and respiratory tract to sample what is happening on the surface (Figure 3a).

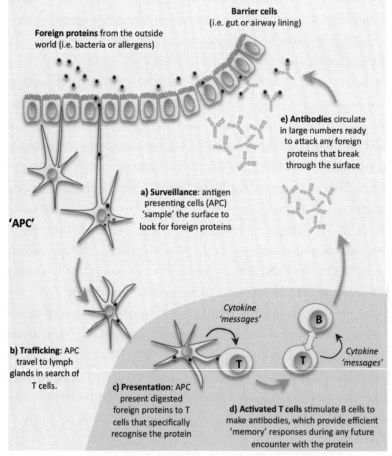

Figure 3   Events leading to a 'memory' immune response

When they come into contact with environmental antigens (including allergens), they 'ingest' them and become activated and ready to defend. Their level of response depends on the level of danger they perceive. It would be counterproductive for them to over-react and cause unnecessary inflammation if there is no real threat. If there is tissue damage, they spring into action producing chemical warning messages called chemokines and cytokines, which recruit other cells to help in the fight.

Once they have taken up antigens, APC are programmed to go back to base in the regional lymph glands (Figure 3b), so they can show the professional immune cells what they have found (Figure 3c). This is what gives them their name, antigen presenting cells (APC). The APC digest the proteins that they find into smaller segments called peptides which they present to the specialised T cells. If the protein/peptides have been seen before, they will be instantly recognised by memory T cells, which will spring into action for an efficient response. But if the protein (antigen or allergen) has never been seen before, then the memory response is initiated (Figure 3d) leading to the production of antibodies (Figure 3e) ready to respond efficiently if there is any future exposure to the antigen.

The APC play an important role in determining the type of response of the memory T cell. The chemical cytokine signals produced by the APC when it presents antigens to T cells directly influence the T cell (Figure 3c). For example, if the APC has encountered a bacterial infection, it will have received very strong inflammatory signals to produce large amounts of antibacterial cytokines including interleukin 12 (IL-12). This IL-12 promotes naïve T cells to develop into Type 1 cells which produce antibacterial responses (see Figure 4 later in this chapter). But if APC do not produce much IL-12, Type 2 allergic-type T cells are likely to develop.

T cells and B cells: partners in secondary 'specialised' defense

These cells are called T cells because they arise in the thymus gland (an immune gland in the chest). Once again, there are many kinds of T cells. Some can attack targets directly, while others help make antibodies.

We have been interested in helper T cells for many years because under certain conditions these are the cells that induce the IgE allergic responses (production of antibodies) by B cells.

There are a vast number of T cells waiting in the regional lymph glands, each designed only to recognise one very specific peptide (=protein part). If a T cell has never been exposed to that protein, the T cell is called 'naïve'. When the APC brings an antigen/allergen for the first time, it will show it to every T cell it meets until it finds one that is designed to recognise that peptide. Once the right naïve T cell is found, it is activated to multiply to make thousands of copies (clones) of itself so they are ready to respond in large numbers if the same antigen comes along in the future. These are generally 'good' clones which are directed against appropriate targets (unlike the rogue clones that cause immune disease).

Once the helper T cells have been activated and matured to produce their own chemical messages, they are ready to fulfill their main function: to help B cells make antibodies to the specific antigen/allergen that they both recognise (Figure 3d). The B cells also expand in number and continue to make large amounts of antibodies, which circulate ready to bind up foreign antigens (Figure 3e). Antibodies are generally Y-shaped structures, which can bind onto various innate immune cells with their 'foot' and bind their specific antigens and the end of each of their two 'arms'. They can also float free, ready to coat a foreign protein so it can be ingested by scavenger immune cells.

The first time we have a particular infection, this process does usually not occur quickly enough to fight the current attack efficiently, but it will provide immunity to the same infection in the future. This is also how vaccines work to provide lasting immunity.

DIFFERENCES IN ALLERGIC AND NON-ALLERGIC INDIVIDUALS

T cells also secrete cytokine 'messages' that tell the B cells what *kind* of antibody to produce. This is where we see further, clear differences in allergic and non-allergic responses (Figure 4).

Helper T cells which produce Type 2 cytokines, including interleukin 4 (IL-4) and interleukin 13 (IL-13), encourage B cells

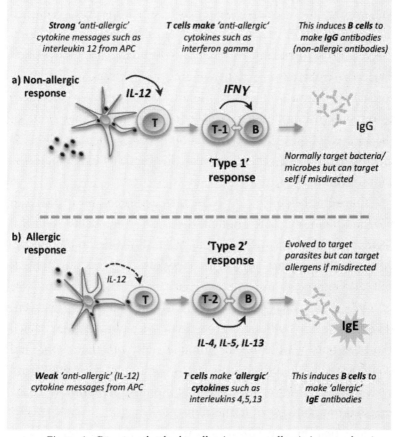

Figure 4   Processes that lead to allergic vs. non-allergic 'memory' immune responses

to produce IgE antibodies that cause the allergic response (Figure 4b). You may see T-helper Type 2 cells also referred to as 'Th2' cells. Although this kind of response has evolved to defend against parasites, when it is directed at allergens it results in an allergic reaction.

In contrast, helper T cells that produce the Type 1 response (cytokine interferon-gamma (IFNγ)) promote IgG production by B cells (Figure 4a). As mentioned before, IgG is the main class of antibody which responds to bacteria, viruses and vaccines. It does not produce allergic histamine reactions.

We are still only navigating in a small corner of the immune universe, but to understand allergy, we don't need to venture much further.

IT IS ALL A QUESTION OF BALANCE

With all that in mind, a person who is allergic to dust mites will have a large number of mite-specific T-helper cell clones that predominantly produce Type 2 cytokines (Figure 5a). They may also have some Type 1 clones, but these will be out numbered. This results in excess IgE production to the mite allergens.

On the other hand, a non-allergic person living in the same environment will *also* have memory clones to dust mite, but these will be mainly producing Type 1 cytokines and not enough Type 2 cytokines to provoke large-scale IgE production (Figure 5b), and hence no allergy to dust mite.

As one response pattern becomes dominant it also functions to inhibit the other. In other words, Type 2 cytokines inhibit Type 1 responses, and vice versa. This reciprocal inhibition amplifies the response in one direction and may be one reason that these 'skewed' responses are hard to change once they are in full swing. Scientists coined the term 'Th1/Th2 paradigm' to describe this model where there are opposing immune effects of skewing the responses in either direction.

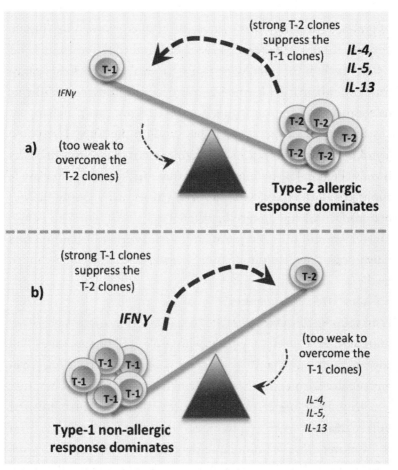

Figure 5   A question of balance between Type 1 (T-1) and Type 2 (T-2) T cells

But remember that these responses are very specific. So a person allergic to mites is perfectly capable of making healthy Type 1 responses to bacteria and vaccines. Although some allergic people may have Type 2 responses to a number of allergens (i.e. pollens and animals) they still have perfectly appropriate Type 1 responses to many other potential allergens which they are not allergic to.

In essence, each response has its own balance.

The 1980s, when these two major patterns of T cell response were discovered, were exciting times for cell biologists. At last there seemed to be a clear model which explained the production of IgE in terms of a Type 2 'skewed' T cell response. There might have been a few holes in the story, but it was the best model so far. It was another ten years before we even recognised another major player in this story. One which had been sitting there in front of us the whole time: the regulatory T cells (discussed later in this chapter).

Although the Th1/Th2 paradigm is now part of a much bigger story, the core observations are still true and have taught us much about immune function. It also inspired us to investigate factors that might alter the balance between Type 1 and Type 2 responses. Only by doing this, did we start to see what was going on at a much deeper level in the immune hierarchy.

So what tips the balance?

Why does the immune system of the same person selectively choose to make a Type 2 response to one antigen but not to another? This appears to be influenced by the local conditions at the time when a particular allergen is first encountered.

A number of factors appear important and these become highly relevant when we think of ways to prevent allergy or to re-condition allergic immune response.

The dose or amount of allergen

There is some evidence that exposure to allergen in tiny amounts is more likely to induce a Type 2 response. Large amounts tend to produce a Type 1 response or to completely dampen any response at all (immune tolerance). This is the rationale for using increasing doses of allergens to switch off an allergic response (see Immunotherapy in Chapter 10).

The route of exposure

As discussed later in this chapter, exposure to allergens through the oral route (the gut) is more likely to induce immune tolerance.

Although this may be partly a dose effect, there is some evidence that immune cells in the gut are more likely to suppress allergic responses, compared with the same kinds of cells in the skin or the respiratory tract. This is the thinking behind the more recent theory that it is better for young infants to eat allergenic foods before they are exposed to them on their skin. In other words, the longer children avoid foods, the more likely they are to become sensitised through the skin. This is completely opposite to the previous allergen avoidance strategies, and is still under research. Another new approach to treating food allergy also takes advantage of this phenomenon: in new studies, children with life-threatening peanut allergy have been able to safely eat peanuts after incremental increases in oral peanut exposure. This simple concept has led to a breakthrough which may ultimately help cure food allergy (see Oral Immunotherapy in Chapter 11).

Exposure to microbial products

Once we recognised the importance of Type 1 responses in suppressing allergic responses, and that bacteria were the most powerful known activators of the Type 1 response, pieces of the puzzle started to fit together. The significance of other observations, like lower allergy rates in children exposed to more infections, suddenly seemed obvious (see The Hygiene Hypothesis in Chapter 8).

In early life, when the immune system is learning the most, it is bombarded with many antigenic proteins from the environment. It does not necessarily see these one by one in an orderly fashion. In environments where there is a relatively higher microbial burden, there is a greater abundance and diversity of bacterial products. APC and other cells in the innate immune system are hardwired to react on contact with these and produce Type 1 responses. If an allergen such as dust mite is first seen in a soup of microbial antigens, it is not hard to imagine why this suppresses any tendency for Type 2 responses.

There has been growing speculation that progressively cleaner living has reduced this natural source of Type 1 stimulation. Exposure to some bacteria, particularly harmless (nonpathogeneic) bacteria, is critical for immune development. Children in highly developed countries not only have fewer bacterial infections, but they also have altered exposure to harmless 'health promoting' bacteria (Chapter 8). Although viral infections are still abundant, these may not provide the same pattern of immune stimulation.

Understanding this allergy protective effect will also be useful in the development of allergy vaccines, and there has already been some preliminary research combining allergens (or their genes) with various microbial products to promote Type 1 cytokines and retrain the immune response.

Other factors that might tip the balance

There are likely to be other factors which can alter cell behaviour, but we don't fully understand these. Speculation still surrounds the possible role of factors such as vitamin D and nutrients with anti-inflammatory effects in the diet, including omega-3 polyun-saturated fatty acids and antioxidants (Chapter 8).

A BIGGER STORY AND A NEW PLAYER

Immature (naïve) T cells can mature to develop into either Type 1 or Type 2 T cells. But a small proportion also develops into another class of 'regulatory' T cells (Figure 6), known as 'Treg'. For many years, nobody paid much attention to this tiny fraction of cells, and the Th1/Th2 paradigm remained the main model to describe the Type 2 skew in allergic disease. But holes started to appear in this simple 'see-saw' model. Not everything could be explained by a simple shift in the Type 1 versus Type 2 balance.

First, it was noted that when immune cells were isolated from the blood of allergic individuals, they often produced increased amounts of *both* Type 1 and Type 2 cytokines when an allergen was added to the test tube. Second, in conditions such as eczema and asthma, Type 1 cells were often seen in diseased tissues alongside Type 2 cells, fuelling the inflammation. These simple observations suggested that there might be a more general increase in immune activity in allergic disease, rather than a simple skew.

The third and perhaps most striking inconsistency was the growing recognition that the immune epidemic applied equally to both Type 1 and Type 2 diseases. This is a good example of different fields of medicine working separately for many years before they realised common ground. For quite some time specialists in the allergy field had laboured under the impression that the modern environment was causing Type 2-skewed immune responses. We were searching for these elusive Type 2 promoting factors. At the same time, in the opposite corner of the immune universe, the autoimmune field was experiencing a surge in diseases caused by Type 1 immune reactions. For them, the modern environment seemed to be having Type-1 skewing effects.

Broadly speaking, auto-immunity describes immune responses directed at our own 'self' antigens (also called auto-antigens) such as the pancreas (in diabetes), the joints (in rheumatoid arthritis), the nervous system (in multiple sclerosis), and the bowel (in inflammatory bowel disease). It was puzzling that some environmental changes appeared to be promoting Type 1 responses in some people but Type 2 responses in others. Even stranger, these opposite responses could be seen in the same person. Although differences in genetic predisposition might explain part of this (see Genetics of Allergy in Chapter 7) there was clearly something else going on.

It was not until the turn of the new century that another theory started to emerge. In both fields there was mounting evidence that cleaner societies and higher living standards were associated with a rise in allergy *and* in autoimmunity. This indicated that these environments were having an effect on immune regulation in general.

Once the penny dropped, many other observations suddenly started to make more sense. In addition to inducing Type 1 responses, microbial products were found to activate cells with strong regulatory properties. They also strongly induce secretion of cytokines such as interleukin 10 (IL-10) that dampen responses. The reason for this became obvious: when you initiate an inflammatory response to kill bacteria, you also need to make sure that your off-switch is activated so the inflammation does not continue out of control. IL-10, which had previously been classified as a Type 2 cytokine in the early days of the Th1/Th2 paradigm, then became re-defined as a 'regulatory' cytokine because of its potent properties as an off-switch. As soon as we started to focus on IL-10, we realised that it was everywhere. Many immune cells were producing it including APC, helper T cells and newly recognised groups of specialised regulatory cells. But IL-10 was also coming from many non-immune cells in the skin, airways and the gut; all the tissues that first come into contact with bacteria and the environment.

In an environment where there are lots of bacteria around, the immune system is on high alert. The products of these bacteria are around all the time without necessarily causing an infection, but they can be enough to provide a constant stimulus to the immune system. So in these environments, the IL-10 system and specialised regulatory cells are more activated to keep control and prevent uncontrolled inflammation. As a result, this special ops 'anti-terrorist' team is also well trained and on high alert for any rogue elements from within. IL-10 and other 'regulatory' cytokines, such as transforming growth factor beta (TGF-ß), play an important role in suppressing both Type 1 and Type 2 clones (Figure 6).

But in cleaner environments, where there is less external

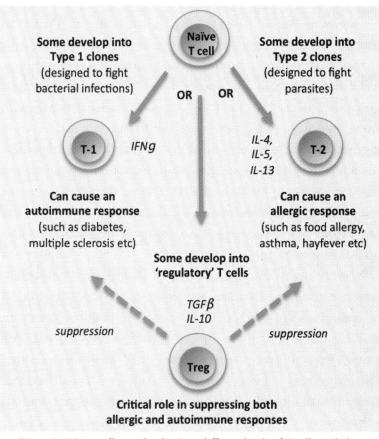

Figure 6   Naïve cells can develop into different kinds of T cells, including
Type 1, Type 2 and Tregs

threat, these squads of regulatory cells do not get the same warning signals. It is proposed that they go off high alert, and without constant training, they get out of condition. This means that they are also less alert to terrorist threats within from any Type 1 and Type 2 clones that threaten to get out of control (Figure 6).

Well, that is the theory anyway. It is the best model so far and seems to better explain why the same environmental changes might have promoted both Type 1 (autoimmune) and Type 2 (allergic) diseases (Figure 6). We don't pretend that we have the full picture yet, but this was a significant progression.

As always, there was huge excitement with this change in thinking, and regulatory T cells were in the spotlight. If these cells that seemed to be so important in controlling disease were failing, could we retrain them to fight disease?

MORE ABOUT MASTER CONTROLLER REGULATORY T CELLS

Regulatory T cells are often nicknamed 'Treg', and by now you will not be surprised to learn that there are several kinds of these too. Some release cytokines, like IL-10 and TGF-ß (Figure 6), to mediate their suppressive effects. Others produce no cytokines at all but have very strong suppressive activity when they come into direct contact with other cells.

One of the reasons that it took so long to realise that there were specialised T cells in the mix was that they look just like all the other T cells. Different classes of immune cells have different surface markers that allow them to be identified. For example, helper T cells all have a marker called CD4 which distinguishes them from other T cells, and when these helper T cells are activated, they also express a marker called CD25. As Treg also express both CD4 and CD25, it is not hard to see why they did not stand out. They only make up a tiny proportion of the total CD4 cells; another reason they were missed.

Over the decades, some of the largest advances in our knowledge of the immune system have come from when it fails. We have learned much from the very, very rare children who are born with mutations in very specific immune genes. By seeing what happens when a gene is completely absent, we can learn a great deal about the function of that gene. That is exactly how we learned more about the function of Treg.

In 2001, around the same time that the allergy and the autoimmune researchers were getting together to focus on regulatory pathways, yet another branch of immunology was making a very interesting discovery. The field of 'immune deficiency' is devoted to studying the effects of missing immune genes. They had just found a very rare fatal syndrome that was caused by a complete failure of immune regulation. In this extreme condition, called IPEX syndrome, babies are born with multiple, severe, autoimmune diseases, including diabetes, thyroid failure and inflammatory bowel disease. They also have an eczema rash. Researchers discovered that this condition was due to a very specific mutation in a gene called FOXP3. This suddenly provided another missing piece of the puzzle.

FOXP3 is predominantly expressed in Treg cells and is the master control gene of their development and function. When this gene is completely absent, there are no Tregs, no control of the immune system and rogue clones completely take over in such an extreme way it is often fatal. So it was this small handful of very sick infants with IPEX who taught their doctors what would otherwise have taken many decades to discover.

IPEX is an extreme example and clearly in most people with allergy and autoimmunity the FOXP3 gene is not defective. Rather, scientists were proposing that it might just be under expressed as a result of lack of microbial stimulation in our cleaner environments.

Once allergy researchers started to look to FOXP3 in their models, they also found a subgroup of CD4/CD25 T cells which also expressed the FOXP3 gene. When these Treg were added to a test tube, they could suppress an allergic response. More importantly, in patients receiving immunotherapy for treatment of their allergy, it was noted that this group of cells became more active. IL-10 regulatory responses were also seen to increase after immunotherapy. This supported the notion that Treg populations can be induced to suppress an allergic response.

It is still early days, and like so much of this story, we don't yet have a universal solution. This voyage of discovery continues, but these events have also highlighted that answers are often found outside our immediate field.

ALL OF THAT IN A NUTSHELL

We might love to discuss all these complexities in detail at our international meetings, but we also make a habit of summarising and boxing the key messages for the audience, and ourselves. We all take great comfort in neatly compartmentalising complex concepts, so I will do that here too. If we acknowledge that it is probably even more complicated than we yet know, we can break down this particular topic into some simple points:

- In the widest sense, two things seem to be going wrong in allergy. First, there is an increased tendency to make Type 2 clones. Second, the regulatory pathways fail to suppress these.
- Environmental changes may be driving both of these processes. Although the cleaner environment underlying the hygiene hypothesis is the most obvious environmental effect that could be doing this, there are clearly many other candidates to be considered.
- Rather than allergy or autoimmunity being due to any specific defects in immune function, it seems more likely that they are due to drifts in patterns of gene expression as a result of environmental changes.

That brings us to my favorite topic: when the allergy story really begins.

6

Setting the scene: the importance of early life

This is my soapbox. And I love every chance I get to stand on it. We all have our passions, things we stand up for and ardently espouse, and this is mine. Most of my research is focused on the early life origins of allergic disease; how allergic immune responses first develop, what might cause this, how we can predict it and, most importantly, how we might prevent it. In theory, the very fact that modern diseases have increased, means that they *must* be modifiable. The same environmental factors that are *promoting* the disease, could also be actively harnessed to *reduce* the risk of disease.

Medicine has traditionally been concerned with diagnosing and treating established disease with a major focus on adulthood. It has taken some time to convince the establishment that the keys to many adult diseases actually have their origins in early life, long before symptoms appear. The message is finally getting through, but the emphasis is still heavily on 'adulthood' and on 'treatment', and we need to keep working to shift this traditional mind-set. The discipline of Paediatrics and Child Health is still widely regarded as a subspeciality area, and its importance is typically under-emphasised in most medical curricula. It might seem obvious to say that childhood is the foundation for *everything* that follows. But that said, we paediatricians still have to continually remind our colleagues working in 'adult' medicine that paediatrics is not a subspeciality, but rather includes *all* aspects of medicine in the most critical period of life: when everything is developing and all structures, functions and patterns of behaviour are established.

We need to remember just how much we have already achieved with preventive measures in early life. On a recent walk through the local graveyard, all of the tiny graves were a solemn reminder of just how high the child mortality was, not even a century ago. With only the black crows looking on and barely a blade of grass, the little graves are marked out in the dusty red dirt by small ornate iron railings. Reading the names of so many infants and young children taken from their families, it was easier to appreciate just how much things have changed. And how much we take for granted now. Simple improvements in nutrition and living conditions have made such a vast difference. Antibiotics have saved so many lives. But arguably the greatest human achievement, ever, in preventative medicine, has been the introduction of vaccines. This simple strategy has virtually eradicated many serious infections such as diphtheria, polio, tetanus, small pox and numerous other potentially fatal diseases from many regions. We may have forgotten the devastation caused by these diseases, because they are rarely seen now. We may also be dealing with a new set of problems. Obesity may have replaced under-nutrition. Allergy, asthma and autoimmunity have displaced infectious diseases. But we don't want to go back to where we were. We need to move forward to find new strategies, new ways of restoring balance and new solutions to the problems we now face.

We know there are many obstacles, but with new technologies we are better placed than ever before to tackle these problems. We still need to spend valuable 'health dollars' on treating established diseases, but we need to invest more of our resources to understand and modify the early risk factors that lead to these diseases in the first place. Prevention should be the ultimate goal, and a much better way to reduce the disease burden. But this does mean holding a long-term vision. And we all have a role to play in keeping that focus. A collective consensus can have an important influence over government and health policies, which are often swayed by shorter-term political agendas.

Among the many crusaders of this cause has been the team from the University of Southampton in the United Kingdom. Their vision[1] led to the formal establishment of a new field of medicine in this area, called Development Origins of Health and Disease, or DOHaD[2] (for a brief history of how DOHaD began, see[3]). This inspired new field crosses all branches of medicine. The first international DOHaD meeting was held in 2001 with specialists from all areas of medicine. I was fortunate to be invited as one of the few lecturers to represent the allergy field.

This shift in focus towards early origins is driven by the hope that early intervention may ultimately prevent many diseases. But before we intervene and potentially cause more problems, we must understand normal processes and how early events set the scene for the rest of our lives.

A NEW FIELD OF MEDICINE IS BORN

The overarching concept behind DOHaD is that events during gestation influence fetal programming to permanently shape the body's structure, function, and metabolism and contribute to adult health and disease susceptibility. During early development, when all systems are forming, they are far more sensitive to the effects of environmental changes. This field provided a new platform for looking at the role of the modern environment in the rise in many diseases, with a much stronger focus on early life effects.

Although these notions existed quietly in the background already, the momentum grew out of studies on the origins of cardiovascular and heart disease.[4] In the late 1980s, the Southampton group observed that under-nutrition during gestation and low birth weight were important risk factors for adult cardiac and metabolic disorders. This concept generated much wider interest in the 'early origins' of many other adult diseases and helped shift the spotlight more towards early life. So what started in the cardiovascular field quickly expanded and coalesced to include almost all other fields of medicine, even psychological medicine, which were all represented at the first international DOHaD meeting in Mumbai, India. It was exhilarating to see so many like-minded experts from so many fields converging from all over the world. Since then, there have been considerable advances in this field, most notably with the emergence of potential 'epigenetic mechanisms' (below) that underlie and may explain the observations and theories behind environmental effects in early life.

INTRODUCING EPIGENETICS: A NEW FRONTIER IN MEDICINE

Epigenetics has become the cornerstone of the DOHaD field. It provides a clear explanation of how environmental changes can affect gene expression and alter early development in ways that can lead to future predisposition to many types of diseases. This is perhaps one of the newest and most ground-breaking frontiers in virtually all areas of medicine. This is a very new field, and one that we will be hearing a lot more about.

So what is it?

'Epigenetics' refers to the mechanisms that control whether a particular gene is switched on or off. When DNA was first discovered, there was great hope that this code would hold all of the keys to health and disease (Chapter 7). But now it seems that the 'epigenetic control' of gene expression might be just as important to how we develop as the actual DNA code itself.

While we are more or less a 'product of our genes', it is more accurate to say that we are a 'product of the genes *that we express*'. We all have many genes that are *not* expressed, or *only* expressed in certain tissues or at certain times. For example, every cell in our bodies has the exact same genetic code, yet a different profile of genes is expressed in different cell types, allowing the considerable diversity between tissues such as skin, muscle, bone and each specific organ type. This is achieved by a complex, epigenetic program which coordinates *what*, *when* and *where* genes are expressed.

The DNA of genes is tightly packed to form the chromosomes that are found in the central compartment of each cell, the nucleus (Figure 7). To fit several meters of DNA (containing over three billion DNA base pairs) into each cell, the DNA must be wrapped around 'histone' proteins, like long thread spooled around a cotton-reel. Histones with their DNA spool form bundles called 'nucleosomes' which look like beads on a string. These are then

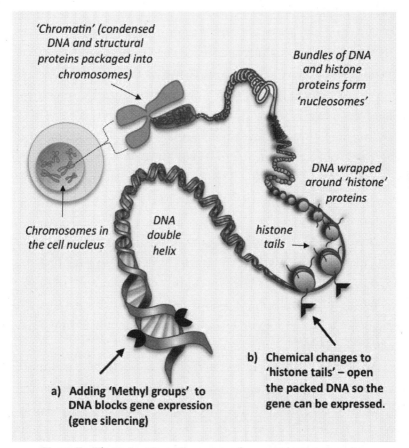

Figure 7   The main epigenetic processes that control gene expression

tightly packed on scaffolding proteins to form each chromosome. This mass of genetic material (DNA and proteins) condensed to form chromosomes is often referred to as 'chromatin'. In broad terms, *epigenetics* refers to the chemical changes that can 'open' the chromatin and DNA structure near a particular gene so that it can be expressed, or 'close' it so the gene stays silenced. For example, the addition of specific biochemical structures to the DNA (such as 'methyl' groups) keeps genes in a dormant state until they need to be expressed (Figure 7a and Figure 8a). Then, when a gene needs to be active and make the protein that it codes for (such as a hormone, a cytokine or a structural protein), the epigenetic program removes these 'methyl' groups so the gene can be expressed (Figure 8b). Chemical changes to histone tails (Figure 7b) can also open the chromatin structure for gene activation. A common example of this kind of epigenetic change is the addition of 'acetyl' groups to the histone tails which opens the chromatin to activate genes (Figure 9).

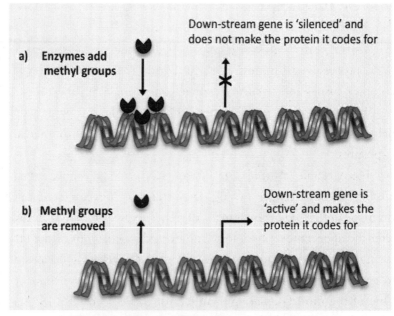

Figure 8   DNA methylation silences gene expression

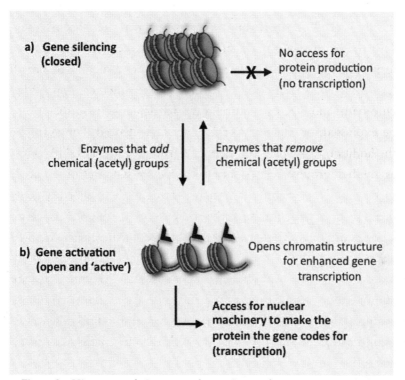

a) **Gene silencing (closed)**

No access for protein production (no transcription)

Enzymes that *add* chemical (acetyl) groups

Enzymes that *remove* chemical (acetyl) groups

b) **Gene activation (open and 'active')**

Opens chromatin structure for enhanced gene transcription

Access for nuclear machinery to make the protein the gene codes for (transcription)

Figure 9   Histone acetylation opens chromatin to enhance gene transcription

During early embryonic and fetal development, these epigenetic processes are highly dynamic allowing so many different, complex tissues and organs to evolve from a single fertilised egg.

The most critical point here is that while the epigenetic program is inherited, it can be *easily influenced* by environmental exposures.

Remarkable animal and insect studies have shown that environmental changes during early stages of development can dramatically change the patterns of genes expressed and radically alter the appearance, physiology and even the behaviour of the offspring. This may be adaptive, and allow the developing organism to alter its development in anticipation of its future environment. One of the most fascinating examples of this is seen with locusts, which can develop into *completely* different forms depending on the

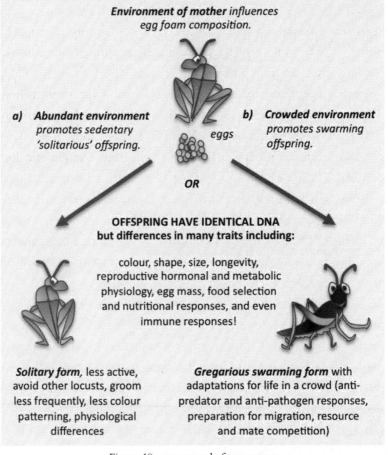

Figure 10 – an example from nature
How the mother can change gene expression in the next generation

mother's environment.[5] Even though they are genetically identical, they look and behave so differently that they were originally thought to be completely separate species (Figure 10).

In times of abundance, when there is little competition for food, locusts are more likely to develop into a sedentary, solitary form (Figure 10a). However, when there is more competition for food, remarkably, a very different gregarious, swarming form develops from identical DNA (Figure 10b). The mother's environment is a key determinant of which form of locust develops because it influences the chemical composition of her egg foam. In abundant times 'solitarious' offspring dominate. However, when the mother experiences crowding and scarcity of food, then the composition of her egg foam changes. This triggers a completely different pattern of gene expression in her offspring, which develop into the 'gregarious' form better suited to the more competitive environmental conditions. The two forms are different in appearance and behaviour, yet genetically identical. This example of nature beautifully illustrates how powerful environmental effects can be, causing completely different development despite identical DNA.

While it takes thousands of years for evolutionary pressures to bring about changes in the DNA sequence, epigenetic changes allow rapid responses to a changing environment.

This new perspective has provided an exciting new insight into *how* recent environmental changes may have brought about such rapid changes in disease patterns. Epigenetics is now at the forefront of many areas of medical research. Identifying how environmental factors modify gene expression to *cause* disease may lead to strategies to modify gene expression to *prevent* disease.

EARLY PROGRAMMING: IMMUNE DEVELOPMENT

During fetal life, the immune system is immature but developing rapidly. Like other systems, it appears vulnerable to environmental changes. It is also heavily influenced by the hormonal effects of pregnancy and the maternal immune system.

The fetus contains many 'foreign' antigens that are inherited from the father. These foreign tissues would normally be attacked by Type 1 T cells (i.e. as part of a Type 1 defense response) which are primed and ready to reject anything foreign. But in pregnancy, complex immunological changes occur to prevent fetal rejection. Some have proposed that hormonal changes actually promote Type 2 immune responses, which protect the fetus and suppress Type 1 tissue rejection. For this reason, some have described pregnancy as a 'Type 2 immune state'.[6] This is still debated and it is far more complex than that. Studies by my research team have shown a that mother's Type 1 responses are reduced in pregnancy[7] but other mechanisms are likely to be more important, including regulatory T cells (Treg) cells in the placenta.[8] But here we can see another example of where 'allergic' Type 2 cytokines can be important and protective without causing allergy.

When I started to work in this area in 1995, not much was known about the early development of T cells in either normal or allergic children. So this became the focus of my PhD, and I was fortunate to work with one of the world's leading cell biologists, Professor Patrick Holt, for three years. The work that we did together[9] attracted enormous attention and was the beginning of my international career.

We firstly found that, at birth, newborn T cells are immature and show a relative Type 2 pattern of response, possibly because they are still under the influence of the Type 2 effects of maternal hormones in pregnancy.[10] Although they are capable of mounting a Type 1 response if threatened by infection, this ability is much less mature than in adults or older children.

Next, I followed the same group of children in my clinic during their early childhood and monitored their changes in T cell function with age. We found that normal children show a gradual and progressive switch to a Type 1 pattern of response over the first years of life, with suppression of Type 2 responses.[11] It was quite a different story in allergic children (below).

We proposed that it was the exposure to the microbes in early life that was important in stimulating this postnatal Type 1 switch.[12] This seemed to fit well with the 'hygiene hypothesis' which was gathering momentum at that time[13] (Chapter 8). We proposed that cleaner environments might be providing less stimulation for this important Type 1 switch, and that Type 2 responses were more likely to prevail and lead to allergic disease. What we saw in the allergic children seemed to support this.

ALLERGY: DIFFERENCES IN IMMUNE DEVELOPMENT ARE ALREADY EVIDENT AT BIRTH

Our critical question was whether early T cell development is different in allergic children. Although signs of allergy are not yet present at birth, there were already hints that newborns who go on to develop disease might already have differences in immune function. One of the most consistently observed differences is in Type 1 responses, which are lower in newborns who later develop allergies. As already noted, Type 1 responses are weaker in all newborns compared with adults, but this immaturity seems to be more exaggerated in allergic children at birth.[14]

Because Type 1 cytokines are important for suppressing the allergic response, it was logical for us to speculate that weaker Type 1 responses could contribute to the Type 2 allergic responses in these children. Indeed, we did see that instead of being suppressed after birth, Type 2 responses persisted and were amplified in allergic children as we followed them with age.[15] This was the first time that anyone had shown this and it was very exciting to have the findings of my PhD published in the leading journal *Lancet*. Even today, this work is still heavily cited by other experts. We don't yet know what is causing these differences, but this work confirmed that abnormal immune development begins much earlier than previously suspected, and even before birth.

In 1999, I set up my own research team to investigate these early differences in immune function in more detail, as well as the factors that could be driving the rise in allergic disease (see Chapter 8). Since then, we have recruited several more pregnancy cohorts, and followed the children so we can to study their immune development with age in more detail. This all clearly takes time, but we are slowly getting more answers.

Scientists are trained to doubt and to question. When we make any observation, we like to see it repeated in independent studies. We like replication for reassurance. And now we have that for the T cell story. My team (under the supervision of one of my senior scientists, Dr Meri Tulic) has used newer technology and once again seen that allergic children show poor Type 1 responses after birth compared with non-allergic children. The allergic children developed an allergic Type 2 response very early, even before they developed symptoms.[16] This makes these early differences in immune function even more convincing.

We have also found that allergic children display differences in the internal machinery of their T cells, with reduced levels of certain proteins involved in the ability to respond to signals.[17] The levels of these signalling proteins are lower at birth in allergic than in non-allergic children; further evidence of an intrinsic immaturity. In our initial studies, the levels of this protein at birth accurately predicted allergic disease.[18] And we have now replicated this again.[19] This might hold promise as a possible predictive test; however, prediction is of limited value until we can do something to prevent disease.

EMERGING DIFFERENCES IN OTHER IMMUNE PATHWAYS

We have just recently addressed another critical question: whether allergic children also have underlying differences in the innate cells. Innate cells, including APC (Chapter 5) are the 'first line defense' sentinels that recognise bacteria and other microbes. They also provide the critical signals that determine how each T cell develops. Without strong pro-Type 1 signals from APC, Type 2 'allergic' responses are likely to develop. Since our early work, there has been strong speculation that this might be the underlying cause of the weaker Type 1 responses to allergens seen in allergic children. Surprisingly, nobody had ever tracked the development of innate responses in normal children, so we did not even know what 'normal' was at this age.

So, for the first time, we have followed children from birth until they were five years of age, collecting blood samples and comparing the innate bacterial responses in allergic and non-allergic children. We do this by stimulating their immune cells in the 'test tube' with lots of different bacterial products, which activate different toll-like receptors (TLR) on the innate cells (Chapter 5). Then we measure how they respond by detecting the levels of cytokine messages that they secrete.

We found some quite striking differences. Normal, non-allergic children showed a slow and steady increase in their bacterial responses with age, and we saw that this closely mirrored their maturing Type 1 responses. This seems to support the notion that the maturation of bacterial responses is linked with healthy Type 1 responses.[20]

But the allergic children showed almost the opposite pattern. They showed excessive inflammatory responses at birth, much higher than the non-allergic group. Then their bacterial responses actually fell with age, so that by five years of age their responses were much lower than those of non-allergic children. So far, there is no evidence that these subtle defects in bacterial defense result in more infections. But they are associated with poor maturation of the Type 1 function, and, just as we had seen previously,[21] they showed progressively increasing allergic Type 2 responses.[22] Clearly, these findings need to be replicated in other populations before we can get too excited, but this adds further to the mounting evidence of early immune 'dysregulation' in allergic children. In the meantime, at least one other group of researchers has seen reduced innate function in allergic children at five years of age, although they only looked at one age group and did not follow them from birth as we did.[23]

Differences are also emerging in other groups of immune cells, including preliminary reports of differences in Treg in allergic children at birth.[24] Although the significance of this is not yet clear, all of these findings support the idea that allergy is not due to a specific gene defect, but rather to a shift in patterns of gene expression in a number of cell types.

We might have previously considered that differences at birth were largely due to the genetically inherited risk of allergic disease, but the concepts of DOHaD have taught us that these differences may *also* reflect the first effects of environmental exposures in pregnancy, and that these exposures may be shifting gene expression to cause a subsequent increase in allergic risk.

IMMUNE DEVELOPMENT IS ALSO UNDER EPIGENETIC CONTROL

One way that the environment might influence the immune system during early development is by epigenetic effects (above). There is now very good evidence that immune development is under epigenetic control. Epigenetic changes determine which cytokine genes are expressed and whether immature T cells develop into Type 1, Type 2 or regulatory T cells.[25]

In newborns, Type 1 immune function genes (like interferon gamma) are epigenetically 'silenced' by the chemical addition of 'methyl' groups (Chapter 5). As infants get older, these methyl groups are removed by the epigenetic program allowing more mature Type 1 immune responses to develop. Development of the regulatory T cells appears to be controlled in the same way. As we will see in Chapter 8, there is now preliminary evidence that gene expression of these cells in the newborn is influenced by maternal microbial exposure in pregnancy;[26] and that this appears to be associated with epigenetic effects.

The rising rates of allergic disease within months of birth has led to growing speculation that environmental changes may be altering early epigenetic control of immune gene expression.[27]

Although this is a new concept, there are already preliminary studies showing that several other exposures in pregnancy can have epigenetic effects on the developing fetus (Chapter 8).

PREGNANCY IS AN IMPORTANT WINDOW OF OPPORTUNITY

Those of us working in the 'early origins' aspect of allergy research are strongly focused on *prevention* as the ultimate goal. Effective prevention strategies mean less people will depend on *cures*. This seems to be a long way off yet, but it is the horizon of our focus.

We *know* that the immune system is being shaped by the modern environment to predispose some of us to allergic disease. By definition this means that the 'pathways of influence' are changeable. So it remains highly logical that, once we understand *what* and *how*, we can hope to use the same pathways to push the balance of risk back in the other direction. At least that is the idea.

Between conception and birth, virtually all our basic structures and functions are formed. The environment can potentially have the greatest effects during this time when systems are immature and more vulnerable. This is also the best time for prevention strategies for obvious reasons, and interventions are likely to be more effective during this period of plasticity before disease processes have become established.

We see allergic diseases (especially eczema and food allergy) appear within months of birth, so prevention must be targeted even earlier, starting in pregnancy. The fact that allergic individuals already have immune differences at birth reinforces this. For these reasons, we look to pregnancy as the ultimate window of opportunity for preventing many diseases. But there is likely to be more than one 'window' for prevention. Because allergic disease is an evolving process, environmental 'drivers' are likely to continue to have effects after birth, so the early postnatal period is another important period for targeting interventions (below).

So far, there are a range of candidate environmental factors which may both 'set the scene' for allergic disease in pregnancy, and then act to perpetuate the process after birth. These include dietary factors, microbial exposure and environmental pollutants (as discussed further in Chapter 8). There is currently intense research looking at how these factors might be influencing immune development, some through epigenetic effects. The hope is that this will reveal the genes that are most vulnerable to environmental effects and how these may be leading to immune diseases. Ultimately, this may help us prevent disease through the same pathways.

THE IMPORTANCE OF THE GUT IN THE POSTNATAL PERIOD

The very early postnatal period is also a critical time for immune development; and another critical time for allergy prevention. To understand how we might promote 'optimal' immune development after birth, the gut is arguably the most important place to look.

Although we used to see the gut as just a digestive tube, we now realise that it is truly an immune organ. It actually houses the largest immune network in the entire body. And this makes sense. This is where we come across the largest amount of foreign material from the environment: from our food and from the billions of bacteria in our guts. We each contain more than 100,000,000,000,000 bacteria! That is more than ten times the number of our human cells. So we are actually more bacterial than human. We live in harmony with these bacteria; in fact we can't live without them. In experiments where animals are raised in completely sterile (germ-free) environments, their immune systems do not develop normally and they develop serious immune diseases including allergy and autoimmunity.[28] This relationship with our gut bacteria has evolved over millennia and there is concern that our modern environment might be disrupting this important bond.

Each infant is born with a 'sterile' gut. In the days that follow, there is a massive invasion of bacteria. This invasion may sound frightening, but it is normal and essential. It stimulates the local immune system and the processes that prevent the bacteria from 'infecting' or 'invading'. A perfect balance develops to our mutual benefit. These friendly bacteria have a home. We feed them. And in return, they provide products that ensure we have a healthy immune system. They also keep less friendly bacteria in check. Everything is happy and harmonious. At least until that balance is sabotaged by an invading pathogen, antibiotics or a major dietary change.

But lately we see evidence of sabotage on a much larger scale. And humans are the culprits this time, not bacteria. Progressive modernisation and cleaner living appears to have altered the balance with our microbial friends. This has been a strong element in the 'hygiene hypothesis' (Chapter 8). There is evidence of changing patterns of colonising bacteria with industrialisation.[29] These differences are already apparent in the first week of life, with much lower colonisation by the important 'friendly' *Lactobacillus* species in modernised countries.[30]

Even more relevant, we see that these differences are linked to increases in allergic disease.[31] Infants who go on to develop allergic disease also have lower levels of friendly *Bifidobacteria* species in the first week of life,[32] and higher levels of pathogenic (disease-producing) bacteria (such as *Clostridia*[33] and *Staphylococcus*[34]). Newer studies also show reduced *diversity* of the gut bacteria in children who go on to develop allergic disease.[35]

Collectively, this evidence strongly suggests that the pattern of colonisation in the first weeks of life may influence the patterns of immune development.

There are a number of ways the bacteria in the gut can influence immune development. These effects also extend far beyond the gut to the rest of the immune system. They promote local protective antibody production and induce specialised APC called dendritic cells (DC) to make regulatory cytokine messages such as IL-10 (Chapter 5).[36] This dampens any tendency for inflammation, which could make the gut 'leaky', and reduces the risk of proteins (from food or bacteria) penetrating deeper into the immune system where they might trigger an allergic reaction or autoimmunity. The DC also influence the pattern of T cell development in the gut, promoting the 'anti-inflammatory' regulatory T cells (Treg) rather than inflammatory T cells (Chapter 5). These cells move into the general circulation where they can maintain the immune balance. Without bacteria in the gut, all these processes break down.

Before we can hope to restore the balance that we have unwittingly upset, we need to known what it was like before, under 'optimal' conditions. But sadly, we don't really understand that yet, and we still don't have clear proof that 'hygiene' is a cause of the allergy epidemic. There are vast numbers of different kinds of bacteria, and many that we have not yet identified. So far, we have made humble attempts to improve early colonisation of the gut using probiotic supplements. Although the initial studies were promising in preventing allergic disease, follow-up studies have had mixed results.[37] However, this is likely to reflect the current shortcoming of our understanding and approach. More research in this area is still ultimately likely to reveal more tangible answers.

The gut is also an important site of other important postnatal exposures such as breast milk, which may be important for promoting 'immune tolerance'. As the main nutritional source for the newborn, breast milk also contains many, many immune factors. These include antibodies and immune cells, cytokines and other nutrients which are important for both protection from infection and for promoting immune tolerance. Breast milk contains substances that promote favourable colonisation of the gut with friendly bacteria. This natural tolerance-inducing food may hold many clues to understanding how to promote tolerance and prevent immune disease in the early postnatal period.

• • •

Without a doubt, early life holds the keys to how and why allergies develop, but it also holds the best opportunities to reverse the allergy epidemic. So, as we consider the environmental culprits that may be driving the rise in allergic disease, we must particularly consider their effects in pregnancy and the early postnatal period.

But before we can further explore how the environment can shape development and our gene expression, we need to understand more about our genes and the inheritance of allergic disease.

7

Genetics and allergic disease

Seeing a small child with an incurable genetic disease die, is one of the most horrible experiences of my career. Part of my job as an immunologist is to look after children who are born with genetic defects that affect their immune systems. For these children a single defect in a single gene is the difference between a normal life and an immune deficiency so severe that even the most innocuous bacteria can lead to a fatal infection. Fortunately these cases are rare, and fortunately we now have the technology to replace the immune system through bone marrow transplantation. But it does not always work, and there are many things that can go wrong.

The happiest moment of my career was seeing my first successful bone marrow transplantation, in a scrawny little boy, who had arrived on our doorstep riddled with infection. We knew we were dealing with an immune deficiency as soon as we isolated a bacterium that does not normally cause problems in children. With obvious signposts in his immune profile, it did not take long to find the genetic defect. He was an only child, so while we were controlling his infection, we searched the register for a donor with the right tissue match. This is critical because without a good match, the healthy immune cells in the donor marrow see the patient as foreign and try to fight their new host. We found one, but the marrow did not take. In the meantime, in a lucky twist of fate, a new baby sister arrived. She was a perfect match. And by the time she was one year old she had saved her brother's life. He is now a completely healthy boy, normal in every way, except that he carries his sister's immune system; a very special and unique bond between them.

We need to hold on to those moments, because it does not always turn out so well. There are times I would rather forget, when no matter what we do, we cannot overcome the effects of the genetic defect. A hundred years ago, when death from infection was so common in infancy, those with immune deficiency were not recognisable among so many others dying of infection. These rare children only became apparent as serious infections became unusual.

As in so many other situations, we discover the true importance of something only when it is missing. Many, many hundreds of genes are necessary for a normally functioning immune system, and defects in any one of these genes can potentially lead to a significant immune deficiency. Over the last fifty years, infants born with each newly described defect, have helped map the genes involved in normal immune function, and helped show the specific importance of each of those genes. This has paved the way for better treatments including gene therapies. Severe immune deficiencies are no longer universally fatal, and survival rates continue to improve. Thanks, in part, to what those critically ill children have taught us.

While specific gene defects have revealed much about the immune system, it has also become clear that asthma and allergic diseases are not due to specific immune defects, but due to complex interactions between our genes and our environment.

It takes hundreds of generations and many thousands of years for the genetic code to change or adapt to a new environment. So it has been obvious from the outset that changes in the DNA code could not explain the rapid rise in allergy. On the other hand, clear clustering of allergies in families also means that genes clearly have some role to play. Certain patterns of gene expression (genotypes) may increase the risk of developing disease, but the disease may not occur unless certain environmental conditions are present.

As with most modern diseases, allergic diseases are due to complex genetic and environmental interactions. In other words, both 'nature' and 'nurture' have a role to play. The very fact that allergies are so common means that the genes that predispose us to disease are very common and must have been there for many thousands of years. Their capacity to promote allergy is merely being unmasked by recent environmental changes.

ALLERGY INHERITANCE PATTERNS: FAMILY RISK

It is widely recognised that children born to allergic parents have a high risk of developing allergy,[1] somewhere around 60–80 per cent risk, depending on which population you look at. But even if both parents have allergies, the risk is still not 100 per cent. This shows that genetic inheritance is not the whole story. When neither parent has any history of allergies, the risk of their baby having allergy is still more than 25 per cent, and this number has been increasing over recent decades; again indicating the role of the environment. While we use a 'family history' to determine the risk of allergy, it is easy to see how inaccurate this is. One hope of genetic studies has been to more accurately predict disease risk and susceptibility to environmental effects, in the hope that disease might be prevented.

THE QUEST FOR SPECIFIC ALLERGY AND ASTHMA GENES

Because asthma has been such a prominent part of the allergy epidemic, most of the early genetic studies were focused on this condition. At the beginning of the Human Genome Project, there was great hope of finding specific 'predisposing genes' for all diseases, including asthma. In 1989, there was great excitement as a team in Oxford found evidence that the predisposition to IgE responses was dominantly inherited within families and that this was linked to chromosome 11.[2] But this was followed by disappointment as other groups failed to confirm this finding. At the time these conflicting results led to controversy and confusion, but they now make more sense with our better understanding of the complexity of gene–environmental interactions.

As with any over-simplistic expectations, it was not long before a number of major obstacles emerged.

A major problem was that asthma is not really a single condition. There are many different patterns of asthma. Even in people with the same pattern of asthma, the pathways to developing disease can be quite different. In other words, the 'inflammation of the lungs' that produces asthma can be the culmination of different environmental factors and many different genes, which lead to that same end result. So far, we have mainly focused on the immune system, but when local tissue is damaged, the function of genes involved in tissue repair are also important.

In the twenty years that followed the first report of a potential 'asthma gene' in 1989,[3] there were numerous reports showing different genes linked with asthma. The main common thread was that the results varied between populations and between environments. So, despite several decades of research by hundreds of scientists, there still did not appear to be any specific genes that were consistently associated with asthma or allergy. Hope of finding one gene to explain asthma and allergy quickly disappeared.

With what we were learning about immune function during the same period, this may be not have been surprising. As we were learning about genes, we were also learning that allergic diseases all seem to be due to environmentally driven shifts in the patterns of gene expression in multiple immune pathways.

While the quest for a gene that causes asthma might seem to have failed, this is not bad news. It is far easier to change the environment than it is to change a defective gene. If asthma were 100 per cent genetic, caused by a 'dominant' mutant gene, then if you inherited that gene from just one of your parents, you would be virtually guaranteed to get the disease, regardless of your environment. One of the best-known examples of a condition with this kind of inheritance is *Achondroplasia*, the common kind of dwarfism. No one who inherits the achondroplasia gene escapes this condition, and no amount of environmental modification can prevent it from developing. We are lucky that asthma is not caused this way.

Similarly, it might also be a blessing that asthma is not due to a 'recessive' gene mutation that causes a specific protein to be defective or completely missing. Everyone has two sets of DNA, one from our mother and one from our father. Surprisingly, most of us carry mutations in some of our genes, but if one gene is not working properly, the other copy can kick in to cover the job. Recessive diseases usually only occur if we are unlucky enough to inherit the same defective gene from both parents. A good example of a condition caused by a recessive gene mutation is cystic fibrosis (CF), a condition that causes progressive lung failure. While there have been attempts to insert a normal copy of the gene into the defective lung cells using CF gene therapy, this has been difficult and disappointing.

Earlier, we came across another example of gene mutation in the IPEX syndrome (see 'More about the master controller Tregs' in Chapter 4*)*. Because this defect is on the 'X' chromosome, it generally only affects males. It is well known that males are more susceptible than females to a whole range of genetic conditions. With two copies of the 'X' chromosome, females always have an extra copy to fall back on. Boys don't. Sorry boys, but this is a department where the girls definitely have the upper hand. In asthma and allergic disease there actually are some gender effects as well (including changes in asthma severity with pregnancy and the menstrual cycle), but this seems to be due to the hormonal effects on immune function, rather than any 'X-linked' genetic effect.

We can make a few summary points about the genetics of asthma and allergy:

- There is an inherited risk of asthma and allergies, but this is dependent on the environment.
- Many genes in many pathways contribute to the development of asthma and allergic diseases.
- These genes may be different in different people.
- It is complicated!

You can apply the same summary for virtually all modern diseases which have increased in the last fifty years!

So if there is inheritance and it is not due to 'defective' or 'missing' genes, how does it happen? The answer lies in a fairly new field of genetics that discovered that there can be several different versions of any particular gene in a population. While these different versions or 'polymorphisms' function normally, their subtle differences can alter disease predisposition.

WHAT ARE GENETIC POLYMORPHISMS?

Each gene is a sequence of DNA nucleotides (the building blocks of DNA) that hold that code for a particular protein. Some changes in sequence can cause the protein to be malformed or not made at all. These mutations cause disease or death and tend to be 'selected out' or be gradually reduced in populations over millennia during the natural selection process of evolution. But very minor differences in gene sequence, which do not greatly affect function, will persist in a population because there is no major disadvantage to having that version of the gene. One of the best-known examples of this is the different 'blood groups' in the population.

Genetic polymorphisms promote the diversity we see in any population, and may be due to only one substituted nucleotide in the DNA sequence. These substitutions are not surprisingly called 'single nucleotide polymorphisms' (SNPs; that we call 'snips').

Not all SNPs produce a difference in the function of the protein they produce, but those that do may have subtle effects, which are enough to slightly change the risk of disease under certain conditions.

Genetic polymorphisms in asthma

Quite a few genes have SNPs that have now been associated with asthma and allergic diseases. Curiously and logically, these are in genes that are involved in the Type 2 pathways, such as IL-4 and IL-13, as well as genes that are involved in recognising microbes, such as a group of receptors called toll-like receptors (TLR) (Chapter 6). These associations seemed to make some sense, given what we know about the importance of these pathways in the allergic responses. In asthma specifically, there have also been associations with functional genetic polymorphisms in a gene that influences the pattern of airway tissue repair after inflammation (such as a gene called ADAM33). Again, this gene was an attractive candidate because of its clear relevance to the abnormal airways repair and scarring in asthma. Yet other SNPs have been associated with difference in response to asthma treatments such as the main 'reliever' (salbutamol) bronchodilator therapy (Chapter 13), highlighting that in the future, treatment may need to be individualised according to genetics.

So, there is little doubt that these subtle functional differences in our genes may alter our risk of disease and our response to treatment. But again, there are still multiple genes involved and these will still vary widely between individuals. Because of the complexity of interactions between different genes and with different environmental factors, measuring a SNP in a particular gene does not currently have any value in predicting disease.

CONTROVERSY TEACHES US MORE ABOUT GENE–ENVIRONMENT INTERACTIONS

When researchers are unable to reproduce each other's results, it makes everyone nervous. Who is right? Who is wrong? It is even trickier when two groups find the complete opposite relationship between certain SNPs and disease. How can they both be right?

This is exactly what happened when researchers started looking at the relationship between asthma risk and certain genetic polymorphisms in a TLR–related microbial recognition pathway (called 'CD14' which is a receptor for bacterial endotoxin). In 1999, research collaborators found that an SNP in the CD14 gene appeared to be associated with an increased risk of allergy in several different populations.[4] While most of the gene sequence

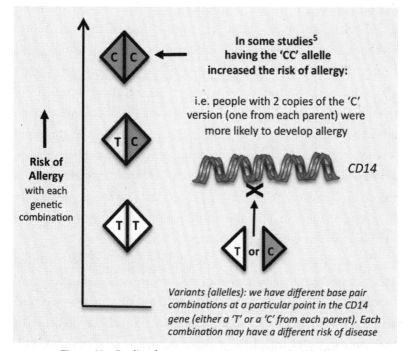

Figure 11   Studies show a gene variant associated with allergy

is stable there is a subtle variation at one particular base-pair (the building blocks of the DNA) that influenced allergy predisposition. Every person inherits either a 'C' or a 'T' from each parent at that site (Figure 11).[5] The varying combinations that appeared were associated with different risk, with the 'CC' combination being associated with allergy, and the 'TT' combination being protective (Figure 11). Since then, several other groups have also seen this relationship, mainly in westernised populations.[6]

However, in 2000, not long after the first report, another group showed virtually the opposite relationship (Figure 12)[7] in a population living under more traditional environmental conditions.[8] In their study, they observed that the 'TT' combination was *more* likely to be associated with allergy.

This seemed to be a direct contradiction and was clearly confusing not only to the researchers, but also to the many readers faithfully following the journal publications in the hope

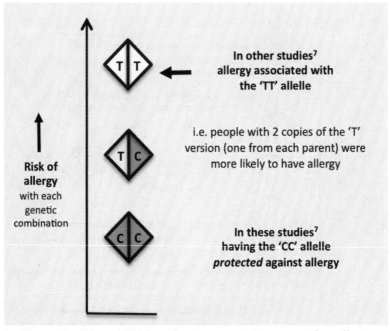

Figure 12   Other studies show the same gene variant protects from allergy

of understanding this field better. Many were rapidly loosing faith that genetic studies would yield answers to the allergy story. But rather than throwing their hands up in despair, the researchers decided to look further.

It turns out that both groups were right, and when their conflicting stories were added together, a bigger, more interesting picture, emerged. They had been looking at two sides of the same equation, which makes more sense when they are joined on the same page (Figure 13).[9]

Once we look at the environment in this equation, it all makes sense. Several new studies examined the same gene relationships in a range of environmental conditions and found that the genetic inconsistencies could be explained by differences in the microbial

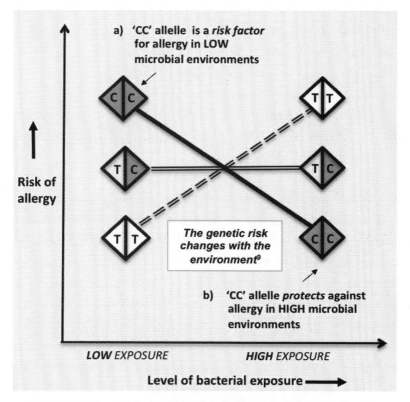

Figure 13 Genetic inconsistencies explained by environmental differences

exposure (Figure 13). The observation that the 'CC' allele was associated with increased risk of allergy was confirmed in children living in *low* microbial environments, is consistent with the early reports (Figure 13a). But the same 'CC' allele was associated with allergy protection (a decreased risk) in children in *high* microbial environments (Figure 13b).[10]

This clearly shows that the effects of some genes can depend entirely on the environment we are raised in. And it is equally true that the effect of the environment will also depend on the genes that we have. There are now many other examples of this kind of interaction with other genes and other environmental factors.

So everyone was right. Everyone was relieved. And we learned something new: unless we look at genetic and environmental factors *together*, we will miss important relationships. It might seem obvious to do this, but for many years these areas of research had operated fairly separately. When I started my PhD in the 1990s there seemed to be two main camps looking at the causes of asthma and allergic disease; those studying 'genetics' and those studying the 'environment'. If you are wondering, I was groomed in the 'environment' camp. But we are learning not to think separately now!

To understand all these complex interactions, we will need the help of mathematicians more and more. With so many genes and so many environmental factors, the kinds of mathematical models that are needed to explore relationships and networks are getting progressively more complicated. This will be yet another example of how we need to enlist the help of people working outside our usual field to solve complex problems. This can also provide fresh perspectives and thinking 'outside the box'. We have had the technology to study these things for a while now, but to take this forward we need international consortiums with the capacity to collect and analyse vast amounts of data using complex mathematical models. Now that this is starting to happen, it is revealing the beginning of what promises to be another very interesting journey.

THE GENETICS OF FOOD ALLERGY AND ECZEMA

Just as for asthma, there is also a clear genetic element to other specific allergies such as food allergy and eczema. This is clear when we look at twin studies. If one twin has food allergy there is a very high chance (over 60 per cent) that the other twin will also have food allergy, but only if they are identical. If they are non-identical twins, there is a less than 10 per cent chance. But notice that even the identical twins don't have 100 per cent concordance; further evidence that the environment must play an important role.

There are also clear associations between food allergy and eczema risk. Both of these conditions have been implicated with altered permeability of the gut, and there is much interest in predisposing genes. One of the biggest recent breakthroughs in understanding eczema has been the recognition that this may, at least in part, be due to 'altered barrier function' of the skin (Chapter 12). In other words, the skin is more permeable than usual, allowing allergens from the environment to penetrate the skin and induce an allergic response. There is also speculation that this could contribute to other allergic conditions such as food allergy and asthma, but this is yet to be proven.

Research in this area has led to the recent discovery of a gene called Filaggrin (FLG) which is very important for skin integrity and barrier function. Mutations of this gene can cause loss of gene function and defects in the skin barrier. Several studies have now shown that some FLG mutations are associated with increased risk of eczema. Studies are now underway to see if the same mutations are also associated with food allergy.

Understanding this new pathway could also provide new avenues for predicting, preventing and treating these diseases. As with asthma, there are also many other genes under investigation for these conditions, which will shed further light on individual differences in disease predisposition.

INDIVIDUALISED PREVENTION/INDIVIDUALISED TREATMENT

The complex interactions between the environment and our genes present another clear question: how does this relate to the treatment and prevention strategies that we use. Do their effects and their effectiveness also vary between individuals, according to our genetic polymorphisms?

Practically everything we use to treat disease comes from the environment, including pharmaceutical medications, herbal and natural remedies. Even lifestyle strategies, such as our dietary choices, are environmental. There are now known to be genetic polymorphisms in many of the metabolic pathways that process dietary nutrients as well as medications. Some, but not all of these, have been associated with subtle differences in individual responses to treatment.

One good example that relates to allergic disease is a genetic polymorphism that can influence responses to asthma medications in some individuals. Subtle variations in the receptor for common asthma 'reliever' medications (such as inhaled salbutamol) can alter the responsiveness to the medication. Again, this effect is seen in some populations but not in others.

When we come to dietary and lifestyle factors that might influence allergy risk, there are also genetic polymorphisms, which could foreseeably alter the effects of probiotics (friendly gut bacteria) and omega-3 polyunsaturated fatty acids (such as fish oil) which are being explored for allergy prevention. There are many more examples. But one of the most important recommendations for asthma prevention is to avoid cigarette smoke in pregnancy and after birth. It is also now evident that certain genetic polymorphisms may amplify the risk of disease in some children exposed to cigarette smoke.

This tells us that treatment and prevention strategies cannot be expected to be 'one size fits all', and that the same strategies are unlikely to work with equal effectiveness in everyone. It also means that we are moving towards a future where we may be able to 'individualise' treatment and, even better, 'individualise' prevention of diseases. But that is a way off yet.

8

The environmental suspects in the allergy epidemic

I might look like a city girl. I have adapted well. But I was born in the middle of the Australian outback, and that harsh but beautiful landscape is where I feel most at home. That is where I like to spend my weekends whenever possible. It is the perfect place to see the wonder and balance of nature and, equally, the consequences when that delicate harmony is disturbed. It does not take much. Nowhere is the resilience of nature more apparent than in the Australian bush, but once a tipping point is reached, the effects can be catastrophic. Out of my window the distant rolling hills might look beautiful in the golden sunset, but I know that they are denuded and may never recover from clear-felling by the well-intentioned many decades ago. But as I look in the other direction down across the valley below, I am glad to see the large tracts of native woodland where conservation has won out over encroaching agriculture, and where farmers work more actively to preserve the environment. Home to many endangered species, we have done our best to restore and preserve our part of the landscape in its natural state with the help of environmental conservation experts. It is probably still far from how it was before the first European settlers came, and it may never be possible to completely restore it and recover species that have been lost forever. But it has found a new balance. Humans might have caused the disruption through ignorance, but the most important thing is that humans are now actively and consciously committed to solving the problem. I can see the dramatic change in awareness and attitude since I was a child. Now, even school children are environmentally aware and learning to care for the environment. As a more interconnected global community, there is a growing desire to look after our planet.

All of this requires an understanding of the environment, and an understanding of our impact on it. My research, and that of others like me, is to take this further and understand how these environmental effects extend to impact on our own health. Humans might not be anywhere near the endangered species list yet, but the modern environmental changes are clearly having an impact on our immune systems. It is all interconnected. We might be the perpetrators, but we are also part of the environment and victims of our own ignorance. But through greater understanding, we also have the power to find the solutions.

• • •

A large part of my research program focusses on the specific environmental changes that might be implicated in the allergy epidemic. My team of senior scientists, clinical fellows, research assistants, nurses and a steady stream of PhD students, has examined the effects of common exposures such as microbial exposure, dietary changes and environmental pollutants; all likely suspects as well as possible candidates in preventing disease. And there are other teams like ours around the globe, now joining forces to discuss this problem.

Environmental change is the only explanation for such a rapid increase in disease over such a short period of time. It has been clear for decades that allergic disease is associated with a more 'western' lifestyle. One of the best examples of the effects of westernisation was seen in Germany in the late twentieth century. Separated under communist rule, former East Germany was sheltered from the rise in allergy rates that were seen in most of the western world, including former West Germany.[1] This was very good evidence that a genetically similar population living side by side could have very different allergy rates if the environment was different. Even more convincingly, when the nation was reunited and former East Germany adopted a western lifestyle, allergy rates quickly rose to equal that of the West within ten years.[2] There are many more examples like this. All of them seem to be linked to changes in lifestyle, diet and living standards.

THE PRIME SUSPECTS

One of our biggest challenges is that with so many complex changes in the way we live, it has been hard to pinpoint the culprits.

But we do have a few likely suspects and it does seem likely that more than one factor is implicated. The best candidates are environmental changes that *also* have known effects on the developing immune system. Our biggest leads are with factors such as changes in microbial exposure, diet, environmental pollutants and a more sedentary 'indoor' lifestyle (reducing both physical activity and vitamin D levels). But even then, the effects of many of these 'suspects' has been gradual and subtle enough to make the case difficult to prove. Although we remain very suspicious of all of these, the current evidence against most of them is still 'circumstantial' at best.

THE HYGIENE HYPOTHESIS

The best-known and most popular theory used to explain the allergy epidemic is the 'hygiene hypothesis'.[3] This proposes that declining exposure to bacteria and microbes may be predisposing us to allergic immune responses. There is no doubt that treatment and prevention of bacterial infection has been a major medical advance. Less than a century ago high proportions of children still died of infection and many of their mothers died of 'childbirth fever'. Better sanitation, vaccination and antibiotics have saved millions of lives, and improved our quality of life and life expectancy. But there has been growing speculation that our cleaner environment may come at a cost, and may be contributing to the rising rates of both allergy and autoimmunity (Chapter 4). The evidence for this 'case against hygiene' comes from both laboratory experiments and population studies.[4]

In populations we can observe trends or associations that are suggestive of this change, but which are difficult to prove causally. But the case is strengthened when we see the same patterns over and over. Early childhood experiences that may be associated with *higher* microbial exposures include attendance at child-care (or other frequent exposures to other small children), having older siblings who 'bring home' infections, having pets who carry microbes and/or living in close proximity to animals on farms. These factors have been shown to protect from allergic disease in many studies. Conversely, factors that might be associated with *lower* early microbial burden, such as caesarean rather than vaginal birth, use of antibiotics, and minimal exposure to older children and animals have all been linked with increased risk of developing allergic disease. Although these associations are indirect and the level of *actual* microbial exposure was not measured in many of these studies, the circumstantial evidence generally points in the same direction: lower microbial exposure is associated with higher rates of allergic disease.

The hygiene story originally focused on 'infectious' microbes. Because these cause illness and disease, their effects are far more obvious, and there is very good evidence that the rates of most infectious diseases has declined.[5] However, the role of these microbes may be less important than the friendly 'non-pathogenic' bacterial microflora we are exposed to every day in far greater numbers. The largest exposure to non-pathogenic bacteria occurs in our intestines, where they play an integral role in immune development and gut function. We have actually evolved to have a symbiotic or mutually beneficial relationship with these bacteria. This has led to concerns that environmental change may be disturbing this fine balance and that it is affecting our immune function. In support of this idea, studies have shown differences in the early gut bacteria of babies born in western countries, such as Sweden, compared with less developed regions, such as nearby Estonia when it was a former Soviet state.[6] And it may be no surprise that allergy rates were much higher in Sweden at that time. This shifted the spotlight to the critical role of friendly 'non-pathogenic' bacteria in the hygiene hypothesis.

Animal studies add stronger, more direct evidence of the allergy-protective effects of bacteria. One very famous study showed that mice who were born and raised in a 'germ free' environment did not develop normal immune function.[7] As we began to see in Chapter 5, the gut houses the largest immune network in the body. Enormous numbers of immune cells normally move about beneath the gut lining and within the closely associated lymph glands. In the 'germ-free' animals, these immune networks did not develop properly, and as a result the animals were prone to both allergic and autoimmune diseases. Although adding bacteria to their environment could generate normal immune function, this depended on the age of the animal and was only possible in very young animals. In other words, there was 'a point of no return', after which the immune system could not recover; again highlighting the importance of critical windows in early life. This study gave very compelling evidence that normal colonisation of the gut by non-pathogenic bacteria is essential for normal immune maturation. Obviously, in humans, even our western environment is not germ free, but it is likely that more subtle changes in our microflora could be having effects on immune function. As noted earlier, new human studies also support the theory that there is a reduced level of 'diversity' in the species of bacteria in the guts of allergic children.[8]

Other animal studies show that *giving* bacteria can suppress allergic immune responses, by promoting 'regulatory' cells and Type 1 immune cells which both can suppress the allergic Type 2 response. Not only can microbial products suppress allergy in animals who already have allergic symptoms, but they can also prevent the development of allergy in offspring when given to pregnant animals.[9] Some studies are beginning show bacteria can have 'epigenetic' effects (Chapter 6) on immune gene expression. The closest we have come to allergy prevention with bacteria in humans is using probiotic bacteria. Although there was early promise with these studies, the effects are still inconclusive (Chapter 9). This may be because adding a single strain of probiotics is like adding a single drop to the vast ocean of gut bacteria. There are at least ten times more bacteria inside our intestines than there are human cells in our entire body. If it comes down to a cell count, we are more bacterial than human. It is hardly surprising that these bacteria can have a huge effect on our health and bodily functions.

So, while there is little doubt that early gut colonisation is essential for normal immune development, we still have much to learn about the vast and complex microbial world that exists inside each of us. This world has been almost as elusive as exploring deep space. There are some gut bacterial strains that are well known to us, but there are many more that we have only just had glimpses of, and even more that we have not yet discovered. We do know that there are wide individual variations in bacterial profiles, and that we each carry a pattern like a 'fingerprint', which stays fairly stable throughout our lifetime. This seems to be a product of our early life events. If we can understand what patterns of colonisation are 'optimal' and how we can achieve these profiles, we may be able to develop better strategies to prevent immune disease. Even so, changing microbial exposure is likely to be one of many other environmental exposures contributing to the allergy epidemic.

THE ROLE OF VIRAL INFECTIONS

Despite the declining burden of bacterial and parasitic infections, we are still plagued by common viruses. In fact, viral infections are now the most common cause of acute illness in childhood. Viral chest infections are one of the strongest risk factors for allergic airways disease (asthma), although the complexity of this relationship has been difficult to dissect. Wheezing lower respiratory infection in the first year of life is a powerful risk factor for asthma by school age.[10] This strongly suggests that viral-induced lower airway inflammation during this early period can have profound long-term effects, which are greater than the effects of inflammation at later ages.[11] This may be due to tendencies of viruses to promote Type 2 'allergic' responses,[12] even more so at this age when Type 1 immune function is less mature.[13] Furthermore, if allergy is already present, wheezy chest infections appear to hugely amplify the risk of developing asthma.

To complicate this further, there is also evidence that *susceptibility* to viral infection and its spread to the lower respiratory tract in young children at high risk of allergy is directly related to their diminished capacity to mount Type 1 immune responses.[14] So it is hard to know which comes first. Is there an immune defect that predisposes to the virus? Or is the virus having an effect on immune function? Or both? What we can say with certainty is that this further highlights the complex inter-relationships between systemic immune propensity and how the local effects of viral infections can be amplified by systemic Type 2 responses, and probably vice versa.

THE VITAMIN D HYPOTHESIS: ANOTHER CONSEQUENCE OF MODERN LIFESTYLE CHANGES?

Another emerging theory behind the rise in many immune diseases is the 'Vitamin D hypothesis'.[15] This is based on a range of observations, including the importance of vitamin D for the developing immune system, and evidence that modern lifestyle changes are associated with a rise in the risk of vitamin D insufficiency. There is also evidence that vitamin D is important for early lung development, and that there are genetic links between genetic polymorphisms (Chapter 7) in vitamin D metabolism and asthma.[16] It is even proposed that there may be links between the gut micro flora and vitamin D, which could together explain the rise in both allergies and autoimmune diseases.[17]

Very little vitamin D is present in food (it only occurs naturally in a few foods such as oily fish and egg yolk) so circulating levels are mainly determined by exposure to sunlight, which is necessary for synthesis of vitamin D in the skin. In regions where there is low sun exposure during the winter months, vitamin D levels vary seasonally, and it is notable that there have been geographical and seasonal variations in immune function and allergy symptoms.[18] It is also interesting that the rate of food allergy has also been noted to vary with the season of birth, in both North America[19] and Australia;[20] again highlighting the potential importance of vitamin D levels in early development. Because modern lifestyles mean more time indoors, more 'screen time' (computers and television) and less exposure to sunlight, there has been concern that relative vitamin D deficiency could be contributing to the rise in the risk of immune disease. Vitamin D insufficiency is now common in a large proportion of pregnant women[21] and newborns[22] in these regions.

There is some evidence linking low vitamin D levels with both allergic disease[23] and autoimmune diseases (such as multiple sclerosis, type 1 diabetes and inflammatory bowel disease[24]).

Because vitamin D promotes 'Treg' activity (Chapters 4 and 5) this is one explanation of how vitamin D deficiency could cause a rise in all these diseases. However, while this is a strong theory, it has not been proven, and there are many uncertainties.[25]

The relationship between vitamin D levels in early life and allergy is also inconclusive and confusing. In some studies, vitamin D intake during pregnancy has been associated with reduced early childhood wheeze,[26] asthma and allergic rhinitis, and eczema.[27] But in others, there was an opposite effect of early vitamin D exposure,[28] so this part of the story is still far from clear. However, this is now an area of great interest and with intense research, there will hopefully be greater clarity soon. There are currently several randomised controlled trials to determine the allergy preventive effects of vitamin D supplementation in pregnancy which will address this question more definitively.

DIETARY CHANGES: WE ARE WHAT WE EAT

All of the building blocks that make up our bodies, and all of the nutrients required to keep us going, come from our diet. We truly are what we eat. So changing dietary patterns are another obvious place to look in our search for a culprit in the allergy epidemic. There have been major changes in our dietary patterns,[29] and this is a large focus of research in my group.[30]

Modern diets differ in many respects from more traditional diets. We eat much more complex, processed and synthetic foods and far less fresh fish, fruits and vegetables. As a result, there have been many changes in the intake of various dietary components including various antioxidants, vitamins, and omega 3 polyunsaturated fatty acids (n-3 PUFA). Most of these factors have been shown individually to have effects on immune function, but again, because of the complex changes in diet, it remains difficult to attribute the rise in allergies to any one factor.[31]

The role of falling intakes of omega-3 fatty acids?

One of the most significant dietary changes with progressive urbanisation has been declining consumption of anti-inflammatory omega-3 polyunsaturated fatty acids (PUFA) and increasing intakes of more inflammatory saturated fat, synthetic fats and omega-6 PUFA. Today, in western diets, intake of omega-6 PUFA (from products such as margarines and vegetable oils) is more than twenty times the intake of omega-3 PUFA (from foods such as oily fish). This is dramatically higher than in traditional diets in which omega-6 PUFA and omega-3 PUFA were approximately equal. The flow-on effect of this is that child-bearing women have lower omega-3 PUFA levels in pregnancy and lower levels in breast milk with higher levels of n-6 PUFA. This means that the fetus and young infant are exposed to a more inflammatory fatty acid profile, leading to concern that this may be contributing to the growing risk of inflammatory immune diseases such as allergy.

In support of this theory, a series of studies have observed that lower consumption of oily fish in pregnancy[32] and early childhood[33] is associated with greater risk of asthma and allergic diseases. This is consistent with the known effects of omega-3 PUFA: laboratory studies show these fatty acids suppress inflammatory responses of many immune cells including T cells.[34]

This knowledge led to the first allergy prevention study to use fish oil in preschool children. Disappointingly, starting fish oil supplements at around six months of age did not prevent later allergies.[35] More recently, we undertook a similar study, but started the fish oil supplement much earlier, immediately after birth, to see if this might be more successful. Unfortunately this too had no effect[36] fuelling speculation that *if* fish oil is to have *any* benefit, it would be more likely to be earlier still; in utero.

The role of my research team in this story actually began well before this, when we began by looking at the effects of giving fish oil in pregnancy. In 1999 we started the first maternal supplementation study looking at the immune effects of fish oil on the fetus. Dr Jan Dunstan took on this project as my first PhD student. She recruited almost 100 women who received high dose fish oil (or a placebo) from twenty weeks gestation.[37] We saw a significant increase in the omega-3 PUFA levels in the cell membranes of the newborn babies whose mothers had been on fish oil.[38] This confirmed that the maternal supplement changed the fatty acids levels in the fetus. Next we showed that the fish oil group had a lower level of Type 2 'allergic' cytokine IL-13 in the infant cord blood at birth.[39] We also saw that higher omega-3 levels were associated with reduced infant T cell responses to allergens[40] and reduced metabolic 'stress' products.[41] Finally, although this study was not designed to prove an allergy prevention effect (which would need a much larger study group) we did see trends that suggested allergy protection. There were trends for lower food allergy, recurrent wheeze, persistent cough, diagnosed asthma, angioedema, and anaphylaxis, compared to the control group.[42] Children in the fish oil group were also three times less likely to have a positive allergy skin prick test to egg at one year of age.[71] We could conclude that fish oil had immune effects when given in pregnancy, and there were preliminary benefits on symptoms that justified further and larger long-term studies.

Since then there have been several other studies which appear to support our findings that maternal fish oil supplementation can reduce the development of allergic symptoms in infants,[43] including one of the largest studies yet (of over 700 mothers) by our collaborating partners in Adelaide.[44] We have also shown that fish oil can increase the level of a specific T cell marker that we identified as protective against allergic disease.[45]

All of these findings are encouraging, and at the time of writing this, we are still awaiting the results of all these studies to be analysed together to determine if there is enough of an overall benefit to recommend fish oil (or more specifically an omega-3 rich diet) for allergy prevention. Even if we do see overall protective effects, it is likely that these will be subtle and, in many individuals, may not be strong enough to overcome the collective environmental pressures promoting allergic disease.

The role of declining antioxidants?

Antioxidants such as vitamin C, vitamin E, selenium and carotene are important for counterbalancing the potentially harmful effects of metabolic byproducts and other factors that can damage cells through 'oxidative stress'. Reduced antioxidant capacity can lead to unwanted inflammation and cell damage. Theoretically, this kind of 'stressed' tissue environment could affect the pattern of T cell development and alter the risk of allergic disease. However, the exact relationship to allergic disease is unclear and this is not helped by two opposing theories, which further highlight the uncertainty in this area.[46]

The dominant theory has been that declining intake of anti-oxidant-rich foods such as fresh fruits and vegetables is implicated in the rise in allergic disease, by adversely increasing susceptibility to oxidative stress and allergic inflammation. There are several sources of evidence to support this. Many animal studies show that antioxidant supplementation can reduce an established allergic response, and even help prevent allergic response when given before an animal is exposed to allergens. In humans, higher levels of antioxidant intakes in pregnancy have been associated with protection from infant allergic conditions, but not all studies support this. Laboratory studies show that increasing the levels of antioxidants in the test-tube can shift the immune response from an allergic (Type 2) to a non-allergic (Type 1) pattern.[47] They can also promote Treg.[48] But the effects in the body on the intricate immune networks are likely to be much more complicated than the effects on single cell types in laboratory experiments. Even when we measure vitamin levels in the blood, we may not be capturing the levels in actual tissues or accounting for different levels of oxidative stress.

However, while levels of some antioxidants have declined, there is evidence that others (namely vitamin C) have actually increased with the introduction of antioxidant-enriched foods, leading some experts to speculate that this is contributing to the rise in allergic disease. This alternative theory is also based on the fact that some antioxidant-rich oriental herbal remedies suppress Type 1 immune responses in the test tube, thereby suggesting they could cause increased allergic Type 2 development.[49]

Ideally, if there are effects, the best time to target prevention strategies is in pregnancy. And the best way to prove an effect is to perform controlled trials comparing allergy levels in volunteers supplemented with antioxidants to those who receive only a 'blank' or placebo. However, because of the uncertainty, there has been understandable reluctance to undertake clinical trials in pregnant women, in case there are adverse effects. Until this is clearer, the safest option is to promote balanced healthy diets.

Soluble dietary fibre: prebiotics
This is another hot topic in the dietary story. Dietary fibre and fermentable dietary carbohydrates (oligosaccarides) have many recognised roles in gut health.

First, oligosaccarides are well known for their importance particularly in promoting favourable colonisation,[50] these food ingredients (often termed prebiotics) selectively stimulate the growth and activity of bacteria in the colon, to improve health. They favor colonisation with 'health promoting' bacterial strains such as the bifidobacteria species and many others.

Second, they also have recently been discovered to have *direct* anti-inflammatory effects on the immune system.[51] Oligosaccarides are fermented to form the short-chain fatty acids (SCFA) responsible for these immune effects.[52]

The declining intake of soluble dietary fibre in refined modern diets have raised obvious concerns, and been implicated in the failure of immune tolerance that is leading to the rising propensity for *both* inflammatory and allergic diseases.

The most encouraging evidence for a role of these 'prebiotic' carbohydrates comes from recent trials giving prebiotics to new-born infants. The children who received the prebiotic in their milk formula were less likely to develop allergic disease than the ones who received the same formula without a prebiotic.[53] This kind of approach could theoretically have more global effects on colonisation than adding single strains, as well as the added anti-inflammatory effects. More studies are now needed to confirm this.

Emerging dietary candidates: folate

The discovery that gene expression is epigenetically controlled by changes in gene methylation (Chapter 6) has led to intense interest in dietary factors that can alter this. The spotlight fell immediately on folate. As a methyl donor, folate provides the 'methyl' groups that are used in our bodies' various metabolic functions, including DNA methylation for gene silencing.[54]

In 2008, a now famous animal study showed that giving folate to pregnant mice had significant effects on the offspring, inducing the mouse-equivalent of asthma and allergic immune responses.[55] The study showed that the folate increased the gene methylation and silenced genes normally important for suppressing allergic responses. This was one of the first studies to show that a dietary change could have an epigenetic effect that produced allergy in the offspring. It is very important to remember that an effect in animals does not mean the same effect will occur in humans. However, since then, several human studies have reported that folate supplements in pregnancy are associated with increased rates of wheezing or asthma in early childhood.[56] Even so, these preliminary reports are based on questionnaires rather than actual folate levels, and 'associations' do not prove folate *caused* this relationship. It is far too early to infer that folate supplementation has contributed directly to the allergy epidemic. Folate is currently recommended to prevent serious birth defects such as spina bifida, and it is important that more studies are done before recommendations are changed. There are likely to be many studies on this in the next few years, which will hopefully clarify the story. In the meantime, there is insufficient evidence to make any changes to current practice. This situation does illustrate that we may face difficult choices when an environmental exposure, which protects from one disease, may actually increase the risk of another.

Other dietary factors?
It is possible that other factors in the diet may be implicated in modern disease, but there is not yet clear evidence of this. Food contaminants such as antibiotics and pollutants could have a role but this is unproven. Many people feel that food additives and preservatives may have a role, especially as these are used more abundantly in urbanised societies. But currently a least, there is no clear evidence of this. This is mainly because there is not much research on this yet, which certainly does not exclude the possibility.

• • •

In summary, diet and nutrition have a critically important influence on almost all aspects of development, including immune function. As such, diet remains a very important avenue in the prevention of many diseases. While many individual nutrients have been implicated in the rise in allergic disease, a 'single component' approach will not fully address the 'composite effects' of dietary changes. As we move forward, it is important to recognise the overall complexity of dietary changes in the wider context and the interaction of dietary change with other environmental factors.

POLLUTANTS: NEW MODERN EXPOSURES

Perhaps the best-studied toxic exposure in early life is cigarette smoke. And in this case there is no doubt about the adverse effects. In addition to many other toxic effects, maternal smoking in pregnancy impairs lung growth and increases the risk of asthma in later childhood.[57] Another of my PhD students, Paul Noakes, spent many years showing that maternal smoking also affects immune development of the fetus.[58] Many of these deleterious effects persist into adult life. New evidence shows that cigarette smoke can change gene expression through epigenetic effects[59] (see Chapter 6). Avoidance of cigarette smoke is one of the few unequivocal recommendations for disease prevention: in both pregnancy and after birth.

Other inhaled pollutants such as traffic exhaust particles have also been linked to asthma in many studies. Notably, exposure to diesel exhaust in pregnancy has effects on fetal gene expression (DNA methylation), providing another good example of how environmental pollutants can modify development through epigenetic effects.[60]

There are many other pollutants that we know far less about. Progressive industrialisation has led to many new environmental chemicals that did not exist in traditional societies, including many products of industry and agriculture.[61] These persistent organic pollutants (POPs), contaminate our food water supplies, and include polychlorinated biphenyl compounds (PCBs), organochlorine pesticides, dioxins and phthalates. Though they may only be consumed in trace amounts, these POPs (such as pesticides) accumulate in our body fat over our lifetime, and levels can amplify with each generation. Many POPs have been detected in maternal fat, umbilical cord blood and breast milk;[62] clear evidence that babies are exposed to these during critical times of development. Again, recent studies suggest that many of these pollutants can also induce epigenetic effects,[63] including effects on global DNA methylation patterns even at the low-dose exposure found in the ambient environment.[64]

A high level of these factors can suppress immune function[65] but the effects of low dose contamination are less clear. Because of their 'oestrogenic' effects, POPs have been also referred to as 'hormone imposters'. Animals in contaminated environments have documented feminisation and male infertility along with immune effects. Because 'oestrogenic' properties can induce Type 2 pro-allergic immune responses[66] there has been speculation about the role of POPs in the rise in allergic diseases.[67] There is one study showing that placental contamination with POPs is associated with higher allergic (IgE) antibody levels in the newborn.[68] But it is difficult to prove that the POP levels were the cause of this. Although POP levels are declining with stricter environmental regulation,[69] this does not exclude a role in the intervening rise in allergic disease, particularly as consequences of an epigenetic change (Chapter 6) may be delayed across generations. POPs have also been implicated in the rise of autoimmune diseases.[70] All of this is very difficult to investigate and even more difficult to prove, but we cannot ignore a possible role of these modern pollutants in the rise of modern disease.

RISING RATES OF MATERNAL ALLERGY: DIRECT EFFECTS ON THE FETUS?

Every mother provides the first environment for her fetus. Her immune system directly influences the developing fetal immune function. It is already very clear that allergic mothers directly increase the risk of allergy in their babies; so the dramatic rise in maternal allergy is another compounding factor in the allergy epidemic. In other words, the environmental pressures causing the rise in allergy could be amplified through the immune effects on the mother. Could this be the reason that we are seeing a 'second wave' of the allergy epidemic (Chapter 4)?[71] We are seeing this in the children of women who were part of the 'first wave' of the allergy epidemic. Is this related? At this point we still have no idea, but this could be one reason for the amplifying effect we see across generations.

Allergy in the mother is certainly a much stronger risk factor than allergy in the father.[72] This strongly suggests direct effects of the mother in addition to genetic inheritance. Maternal allergy is also more likely to be associated with weaker Type 1 immune responses in the fetus (which predispose to allergy) than paternal allergy.[73] Our research team has shown how pregnancy changes maternal immune response[74] and that allergic mothers have lower Type 1 responses to foreign fetal antigens compared with non-allergic women.[75] This means that there are likely to be differences in the 'immune environment' experienced by the fetus in the womb, which could influence its patterns of development. We do know that infants of allergic women not only have lower Type 1 responses, they also appear to have reduced regulatory T cell (Treg) function and other differences in immune function.[76]

This tells us that the fetus is sensitive to the 'internal' as well as the 'external' environment during pregnancy. So as we examine the external culprits in the allergy epidemic, we must consider that in addition to *direct* effects on the fetus, these factors are also likely to have had longstanding effects on the maternal immune system over her lifetime, which could compound their effects on the new generation. This possibility still needs further investigation.

STRESS AND THE IMMUNE SYSTEM: ANOTHER LIFESTYLE EFFECT?
We are all familiar with stress. It can take many forms, and the increasing pace of modern life has been a likely influence on our stress patterns. Rising rates of anxiety and depression could be

a reflection of this. But does this affect our immune system as well? Although *direct* links with the epidemic of immune disease are hard to prove, there are well-recognised connections between psychological wellbeing and immune function. We all know that we are more likely to get sick when we are stressed and 'run down'. Indeed, the hormones produced in an acute (sudden) stress response have well known effects on immune function. The same is true of chronic (long-standing) stress. Stress activates the adrenal gland system and increases production of stress hormones such as 'cortisol'; a steroid produced by the body to help body functions cope with chronic stress. This can change the pattern of cytokines (i.e. the immune messages, see Chapter 5) produced by immune cells and can influence the pattern of an immune response. Stress is certainly a recognized *trigger* for an allergy exacerbation in someone who is *already* allergic. But could it also be promoting the development of allergy in the first place? This is a fundamental question, and to explore this we need to look again at early life when the immune system is developing. The effects of stress are likely to begin well before birth.

The rising rates of psychological stress we see in modern societies are also likely to be impacting many pregnant women. There is already some evidence that mothers who are stressed, anxious or depressed have more 'activated' immune cells with more production of inflammatory cytokines. In extreme cases this can change in the cytokine balance in the placenta, altering blood flow with possible effects on fetal growth and development, including subsequent immunity.[77] This has raised questions about whether there may also be more subtle effects of chronic 'everyday' stress. There is speculation that a range of maternal stressors in pregnancy can have effects on many aspects of long-term health in the offspring: including cardiovascular disease, diabetes, obesity, respiratory disease, neurological development and behavioural disorders as well as allergy and immunity.[78] After birth, there is also evidence that a stressful environment can influence the immune development of the infant, even in early infancy.

So while there are still many unanswered questions about the exact contribution of stress to the allergy epidemic, this is likely to be another inter-related factor with recognised effects on immune function. More research is needed to understand this. In the meantime, it is logical that we take every opportunity to reduce stress in our lives, as this is likely to be beneficial to many aspects of our health.

OTHER ENVIRONMENTAL FACTORS

There has been growing interest in how rising rates of non-vaginal birth (caesarean section) might be related to the rise in asthma and allergic disease. The infant is first exposed to friendly bacteria as it passes through the birth canal. Higher rates of delivery in 'sterile' surgical suites and the use of antibiotics during this early period are likely to be additional contributors in the 'hygiene hypothesis'. There are now a number of large studies that show higher rates of asthma in children born by caesarean section.[79] The risk appears higher with emergency sections than with planned sections,[80] which could be due to other factors associated with high-risk deliveries such as more frequent use of antibiotics.[81] Other studies have also suggested that antibiotics use in the first year of life increases the risk of allergic disease.[82]

Other medications have been linked to allergic disease, but again it is difficult to prove that this relationship is *caused* by the medications. One of the most consistent relationships has been with the use of paracetamol in pregnancy.[83] The largest of these studies examined more than 66,000 Danish women and found that paracetamol use at any time of pregnancy was associated with significantly increased risk of childhood asthma.[84] Paracetamol depletes antioxidant levels, and could been implicated in the development of both abnormal lung function and immune function through this pathway. Acid-suppressive medications in pregnancy have also been associated with an increased risk of developing childhood allergy and asthma.[85] While these effects may not be large, they represent potentially avoidable risk factors that require further investigation.

ALLERGENS: INNOCENT BYSTANDERS?

Although we have considered allergens already, it is worth another word here. Not because they have caused the allergy epidemic, but because they were falsely accused for so long. For many years people have tried in vain to avoid allergens from pets, foods and dust mites in the hope of preventing allergic disease, but this has been unsuccessful (Chapter 9).

We certainly accept that these allergens have unique properties that make them likely targets of the immune systems. We could regard them as irritating characters who are most likely to attract attention. But they are not the cause of the problem. It is now generally accepted that other environmental changes are driving the allergy epidemic, and allergens are bystanders (although not entirely innocent). There is now a shift towards actually using/ giving allergens, rather than avoiding them, in both the treatment and prevention of disease (Chapters 9 and 10).

• • •

After considering all this, we are left in no doubt that the modern environment is driving the rise in many modern diseases. But it is also clear that this is extremely complicated and that it will be difficult to separate the effects of individual factors. And we have already seen how the effect of individual environmental factors can vary according to subtle variations each person's genetics (Chapter 7).

Just as there have been genetic studies looking for 'genome-wide associations' with disease, there also need to be 'environment-wide association' studies that go into similar depth. We need to be prepared to look in completely new directions and with new eyes. We will need to team up with mathematicians with serious computing power to look at these complex interactions. New discoveries have already challenged many past ideas, and produced many shifts in thinking. And we need to be prepared for more changes. We need to anticipate the dilemma of a factor that protects against one disease yet promotes another. Nothing is simple in any of the modern diseases that humanity now faces. It won't be easy, but researchers in our field are up to the challenge.

9

The practicalities: current allergy prevention strategies

The most important part of research is applying it and putting 'theory' into 'practice'. This is really the ultimate goal of what we are doing, and the focus of the rest of this book. While progress is steady, the process of research is slow, and sometimes frustrating when we want to see immediate benefits for our patients.

In writing this I was asked to reflect on the challenges and the obstacles that I have had to overcome. There are many. The constant battle for funding every year. The threat to my team, their jobs and careers if I am not successful. The growing difficulty attracting new graduates to research positions, which do not pay anything like attractive industry jobs. The ever-increasing bureaucratic hurdles. And the mounting piles of electronic 'paperwork' we have to trawl daily. All these factors seem to leave less time and less focus to actually do what we want to be doing. The science. And the translation of the science into real solutions.

But when I think of the greatest obstacles of all, I think I face the same things that we all face: the inner battles of fear and doubt. Wondering if what I am doing is making a difference. Worrying that I am not doing enough. Getting too busy to think, plan, invest and nurture. Not having enough energy left for my husband and family. Allowing stress to take hold. Getting sucked into other people's dramas, instead of looking after myself. Seeing friends get sick and die early from job-related stress. It is the same old story everywhere. Instead of technology giving us more leisure, it has catapulted us into hyper-drive. Our lives seem to be accelerating every year, and I am not sure that is just because I am getting older. So I can honestly say that my biggest challenge every day is to remember to breathe! And to slow down. And to focus on being 'in the present moment'. I have my wonderful 'new age' parents to thank for these ideas, and for dragging me along to meditation classes from the age of eleven. I might not have enjoyed it then, but now I am glad I did it. When I do this I can find a real sense of peace. I can immediately regain perspective and I can consciously choose not to let the problems of the day consume me. And it is easy to get caught up and forget. Yes, there are the usual battles of my job. The funding. The deadlines. Trying to convince people that what we are doing is important, when funding and resources are threatened. But what happens, happens. Worrying about it has never helped. All I can do is my best and what I feel is right. Then just let it go. Things always seem to have worked out for the best. It might not always be what I had in mind. But that is usually a good thing too. I am still learning.

• • •

With a firm foundation in the theory of allergy, we can now move into the practical aspects of the allergy story. Once again, the most obvious place to start is at the beginning of life, and to consider what we can currently do to reduce the risk of allergies developing in the first place.

Another of my professional roles has been to review and update national guidelines for allergy prevention, and translate the international research into practical advice for families and health care professionals.[1] In 2008, expert panels around the world convened to review the evidence for allergy prevention strategies.[2] This was driven by a series of studies that suggested that some of the existing strategies were ineffective. In Australia, I worked closely with other experts to review this advice in light of current evidence. This meant many emails, teleconferences and discussions, which culminated in practical advice for infant feeding.[3]

We can ponder all of the research, but where does that leave us in practical terms? Any practical advice for reducing allergy risk must be based on reasonable evidence that there is some benefit. Early recommendations for allergy prevention were based on fairly weak evidence (limited numbers of studies and/or small studies), because that was all that was available at the time. As more evidence comes to light through larger studies, old approaches need to be revised, as with our recent dismantling of 'allergen avoidance' strategies.[4] This again highlights that nothing is set in stone, and recommendations are likely to change further as we learn more. So here we can only consider the current approaches based on the current evidence. I have to admit that this has not been easy with still fairly limited research in this area.

And there is much more to consider than just the research itself. We must also weigh up the *cost*, the *size of a benefit*, and the *level of evidence* behind any proposed prevention strategy.

For example, is it reasonable to ask parents to undertake a costly, time consuming, stressful prevention regime if the benefit is likely to be small and the evidence is weak? Most would argue that this is hard to justify. Yet some of the previous strategies (such as asking mothers to avoid peanut in pregnancy) could be regarded as both stressful and time consuming, with no proven benefit.

We also need to think about whether the recommendation should be made to everyone, or just to the children most at risk. Ideally, we want a targeted approach where we can accurately predict who will develop allergy and design a specific and effective strategy for them.

How good are we at identifying infants 'at risk' of allergic disease?

In current practice, the best we can do is to determine the rough chance of allergy based on relatives with allergy. Children born into atopic families are more likely to develop allergic diseases (50–80 per cent risk) compared to those with no family history atopy (20 per cent). The risk appears to be higher if both parents are allergic (60–80 per cent) as opposed to only one parent. The risk is also higher if the mother (as we explored in Chapter 7) has allergic disease.[5] These numbers are widely quoted, but are very rough, likely to vary between populations and probably out of date; however, they do clearly reflect that with rising rates of allergy, a significant proportion children with no allergic parents still develop allergy. Although biological differences have been documented in allergic children at birth (before symptoms have shown), including higher IgE levels and lower T cell responses (Chapter 6), so far none of these has been accurate enough to develop as a screening tool.

There is still strong hope that we will develop better biological and genetic predictors of allergy, but for now when we talk about 'high risk' children we are still usually referring to children with a first degree relative (parent or sibling) with allergic disease.

How good are our current prevention strategies?

Well, firstly, it is a very short list, and it has been getting shorter as we strike off old recommendations that are no longer justified. The two absolutely unequivocal recommendations are things that we would logically recommend for other reasons anyway: the avoidance of cigarette smoke and the promotion of breastfeeding if possible. And even then, the evidence that they are *specifically* linked with allergic disease is not actually clear (Chapter 7).

Beyond that, other strategies are relatively weak or as yet unproven. But we need to remember that this is still a fairly young area of research and there are likely to be many more developments yet.

WHAT STRATEGIES HAVE BEEN USED AND ARE THEY STILL JUSTIFIED? The first prevention strategies were based on the idea that if an allergen can be avoided completely, an allergic response to that allergen is unlikely. This approach has been unsuccessful, probably because complete avoidance is not possible. Trace amounts are often present and even if the food is not eaten, exposure can still occur through other routes, such as the skin, which is more likely to lead to sensitisation.[6] With the recognition that specific oral tolerance is an antigen-driven process, there is now a shift in focus towards earlier, regular exposure to allergenic foods to promote tolerance (Chapter 6).

But there is a very important distinction to make at this point. Here we are discussing the role of allergens avoidance in children who are *not* yet allergic. That is very different from the situation *once an allergic reaction has developed*. In that case, it is very important to try and avoid the allergen (i.e. egg, peanuts, cats etc.) that will cause a reaction. In some allergic patients allergens are used therapeutically (i.e. in immunotherapy), but this should only be done with medical supervision because of the risks of reaction (Chapter 10).

Previous allergen avoidance strategies that are no longer recommended

1. *Avoiding allergenic foods during pregnancy:* several controlled studies have failed to show that restriction diets in pregnancy reduce the risk of allergic disease in children.[7] This is actively discouraged because of potential nutritional compromise to the mother and fetus.
2. *Avoidance of house dust mites in pregnancy (and early postnatal period):* Stringent methods to reduce mite levels have actually been

associated with an increased risk of mite allergy.[8] This might be because these strategies also reduce protective levels of microbial products. At this point, mite avoidance strategies cannot be justified for prevention.

3. *Avoidance of pets in pregnancy (and early postnatal period):* Several studies suggest that early exposure to pets may actually be protective,[9] again possibly because of the associated exposure to bacterial products. However, this is a complex relationship[10] and most physicians would not recommend getting pets to prevent allergy either. The current message is for prospective parents not to change whatever their pet-keeping situation is!

4. *Maternal allergen avoidance during lactation:* Again, most studies have not shown any consistent benefit of a restriction diet during lactation,[11] and this is also not recommended.

5. *Delayed introduction of complimentary feeding (foods other than breast milk):* For many years, prolonged 'exclusive' breastfeeding has been recommended for allergy prevention. The original rationale for delayed feeding was based on concerns that young infants have relatively immature mucosal immunity and increased gut permeability, which may increase the risk of systemic allergic responses. However, while early allergic disease outcomes are reduced in children who have not been exposed to complementary foods before four months of age,[12] there is little evidence that avoidance beyond four months is beneficial.[13] In fact, avoidance beyond six months has been associated with increased risk of allergic disease (food allergy, eczema, asthma)[14] and possibly coeliac disease.[15] For this reason, in 2008, most experts in industrialised countries recommended that complimentary foods are introduced 'from *around* 4–6 months of age' and that these should not be delayed beyond six months of age,[16] in contrast to previous recommendations.[17] There are some regional variations in how agencies implement this, but most currently recommend 'around 6 months' (to

allow some individual flexibility) and highlight the need for more studies to clarify this. It is important to point out that these recommendations relate to allergy risk. In developing regions where children are at greater risk of infections (and less at risk of allergy) the World Health Organisation still recommends 'exclusive' breastfeeding for at least six months.[18]

6. *Specific avoidance of allergenic foods*: Even after complimentary feeding had commenced, it was common practice to continue prolonged avoidance of 'allergenic foods'. Again, this is another of the old strategies recently overturned[19] in contrast to previous recommendations[20] based on insufficient evidence to support specific delay or avoidance of foods (such as egg, peanuts, nuts, wheat, cow's milk and fish) for the prevention of food allergy or eczema. Notably, although this is based on the current evidence, all expert bodies identified the need for better studies to determine the optimal time to start complementary solid foods, so this is not likely to be the end of the story. We, and a number of other groups, are exploring this in a series of new studies.

Strategies that are currently recommended, at least at this moment of writing (!)

1. *Breastfeeding:* This is recommended and strongly encouraged for the many nutritional and non-nutritional benefits for both the mother and infant.[21] As noted (Chapter 6) there are many immune factors in breast milk that we are still to understand, and some studies suggest that breastfeeding during the period when new foods are introduced may help promote immune tolerance and prevent allergic disease, although this needs to be confirmed.

2. *If a complementary infant formula is required before solid foods are started*: Here there is a distinction based on perceived 'risk' of allergy. In children at 'low' risk (with no immediate family members with allergies) a standard cow's milk infant formula can be used.

However, in infants at 'high' risk (with parents or siblings who have allergies) there is some evidence that 'hydrolysed' formulas reduce the risk of allergic disease.[22] These are cow's milk based formulas that have been processed to break down the proteins which cause symptoms in cow's milk allergy. Both 'partially' hydrolysed formulas and more extensively hydrolysed formulas have been shown to reduce the risk of allergic disease.[23] There are regional differences in the availability of these formulas, and in some countries only 'partially' hydrolysed formulas (usually labeled 'HA' or hypo-allergenic) are made for prevention because they are cheaper and more palatable. Because they are incompletely hydrolysed, these formulas are not suitable for children who already have milk allergies (who need more extensively hydrolysed formulas, see Chapter 11). Generally, soy milk and other mammalian milks such as goat's milk are not recommended for allergy prevention.

3. *Introduction of complimentary feeding:* it is currently recommended that 'solid' foods are started somewhere around 4–6 months. The timing will vary from child to child, according to their developmental readiness and their appetite. When a child is ready, many specialists suggest that parents consider introducing a new food every 2–3 days according to what the family usually eats (regardless of whether the food is thought to be highly allergenic). New foods should be given one at a time, so that reactions can be more clearly identified, and then continued as a part of a varied diet. It is considered that infants are unlikely to develop a new allergy to any food that is already tolerated, if it is given regularly. During this time, breast milk or an appropriate infant formula should remain the main source of milk until twelve months of age, although cow's milk can be used in cooking or with other foods. *We stress that there are no particular allergenic foods that need to be avoided.* In Australia, where allergy is so common, we have aimed our advice at all

families, including those in which other children already have allergies.[24] Some children will develop allergies no matter what we do. So, if there is any reaction to any food, parents should seek medical advice and that food should be avoided until the child is reviewed by a medical practitioner with experience in food allergy. Infants who already have eczema are at higher risk of food allergies. In general, this advice also applies to these children and we encourage a normal diet unless a reaction occurs. More research is needed in this area, and it is possible that this advice will be amended further as more information comes to light.

4. *Avoidance of cigarette smoke:* There is little doubt about this recommendation. Maternal smoking in pregnancy can have many damaging effects, including effects on lung development, immune development as well as many other systems (Chapter 8). Smoke exposure after birth is also a clearly associated with wheezing illness in early childhood.[25] For these reasons, pregnant women are strongly advised not to smoke in pregnancy and, after birth, children should not be exposed to cigarette smoke in confined spaces. Clearly, smoking should be strongly discouraged at all ages in all people.

Future research opportunities

Finally, there are a series of other strategies for which the evidence is still unclear. While these may have potential benefits, the evidence is not strong enough to form the basis of specific recommendations. These are areas where future research might provide new opportunities:

1. *The use of probiotics:* 'Probiotics' are live microorganisms that, when administered in adequate amounts, confer a health benefit. The most commonly used bacterial strains are *lactobacilli* and *bifidobacteria*. As gut bacteria are known to be critical for normal immune development, there has been obvious interest

in probiotics supplements as a way of promoting 'favourable' colonisation. The first study to use probiotics for allergy prevention showed a staggering 50 per cent reduction in the development of eczema.[26] This Finnish study used a probiotic strafin called *Lactobacillus rhamnosus* GG (LGG), and gave this to the mothers during the last few weeks of pregnancy and to the infants for the first six months after birth. Although these children were less likely to develop eczema by one year of age, there was no difference in other allergic conditions (such as asthma, rhinitis or food allergy) or the levels of allergic antibodies, even in later childhood.[27] Even so, this reduction of eczema was cause for much enthusiasm. But the story has grown murky. Since then there have been at least fifteen more studies with very conflicting results,[28] including a German study that tried to replicate the Finnish LGG study, but failed to show any benefit at all.[29] My research team also spent four years looking to see if giving a *Lactobacillus acidophilus* probiotic for the first six months of life could prevent allergies.[30] But all that work showed no benefits. If anything, positive allergy tests were actually more common in the children who had the probiotics.[31] These conflicting results appear to indicate that effects can vary widely with different probiotic strains, and in different populations. As more studies come to hand, the summary literature (often synthesised by pooling the results of multiple studies in what we call meta-analyses) needs to be updated. The Cochrane Database is an important repository of meta-analysis studies, including studies on probiotics.[32] Based on more recent studies, the meta-analysis is already under revision (*Personal communication from Dr John Sinn, ahead of press*) and will conclude that a probiotic containing a *Lactobacillus rhamnosus* strain *may* reduce the incidence of eczema in high-risk infants, but that there are no reproducible effects of any other probiotics. And no probiotics prevent any other allergic diseases. Again, the authors advise caution in interpreting the pooled data because of methodological differences between the studies.

So, while there is good evidence that gut microbiota modulate immune programming and can prevent allergy and immune disease (Chapter 6), the optimal way of achieving this is far from clear. This confusion does not mean that the gut flora is not important. It means that we don't understand exactly what is 'optimal' or how to achieve it. Of the 10,000,000,000,000 bacteria in the human gut, there are more than 500 different species each with a multitude of strains. There are also huge variations between individuals. In some ways, it should not be surprising that giving a supplement containing a single strain (or even a combination of several strains) is like a 'drop in the ocean'. But this is still an important area of research. Strategies with a more general effect on colonisation could have more potential. For now, given the current level of evidence, it is not appropriate to specifically recommend probiotics for the prevention of any allergic conditions.

2. *The use of prebiotics:* The term 'Prebiotics' is used to describe soluble dietary fibre fermented by gut bacteria. These non-digestible carbohydrates are essentially 'food' for our gut bacteria and can selectively stimulate the growth of beneficial bacteria in the colon (i.e. the *lactobacilli* and *bifidobacteria* species). Prebiotics are present in breast milk and may also play a role in promoting early colonisation (Chapter 8). The fermentation products of prebiotics can also have anti-inflammatory effects.[33] For these reasons, there have been concerns that declining dietary fibre in modern diets might also be contributing to the rising rates of inflammatory and allergic diseases. Prebiotic carbohydrates supplements could theoretically stimulate a more diverse range of 'friendly' bacteria, and therefore be more effective at promoting the necessary diversity than just adding a few strains of probiotic bacteria. There has now been one very

promising study to suggest that prebiotics mixtures added to infant formulae can reduce the development of allergic disease.[34] Infants who received the prebiotic mix had much higher colonisation with *bifidobacteria* compared with the infants who only received a placebo ('dummy') mix. They also had less eczema by six months[35] and over the first two years of life.[36] This was a very exciting finding, and it has naturally shifted some of the enthusiasm from *pro*biotics to *pre*biotics. However, and as always, more studies are needed. The first probiotic studies were equally promising, but we have seen from subsequent studies that it is never that simple. There is certainly not enough evidence to make any specific recommendations apart from breast milk, which naturally contains prebiotics. For now we have to wait with cautious optimism to see how the prebiotic story evolves.

3. *The use of fish oil and omega-3 fatty acids:* Omega-3 PUFA have anti-inflammatory effects, and many researchers have observed that fish consumption or omega-3 PUFA levels in pregnancy and childhood can protect against allergic disease.[37] However, these observations need to be supported by 'double blinded randomised controlled trials' to provide the level of evidence required to make clear recommendations. Such trials use placebo 'dummy' capsules to try to eliminate any bias. So far, there are relatively few of these of large enough size to be conclusive. What we can say is that giving fish oil supplements *after* birth does not seem to have an effect, and that *if* there is an effect, it appears to be more likely in pregnancy. Several controlled trials show reduction in some allergic symptoms in infants of mothers who took fish oil supplements[38] although not all of these were originally designed for this purpose. The largest and potentially most definitive study is being conducted in Adelaide, Australia (with supplementation of more than

700 women in pregnancy).[39] We all hope that this will provide clear direction for dietary recommendations in allergy prevention. For now, it is premature to recommend fish oil supplementation during pregnancy as a preventative measure against allergic disease.

4. *The role of other dietary factors and dietary supplements:* As discussed in more detail in Chapter 8, there are many dietary elements with immune effects that could have a future role in allergy prevention (including vitamin D, antioxidants, folate and other vitamins). However, none of these is anywhere near the stage of making specific recommendations, beyond promoting a healthy, balanced diet. We can say that diet is a critical influence on early immune development and this should remain a research priority.

5. *The avoidance of other pollutants:* A number of indoor and outdoor pollutants have been associated with allergic diseases, particularly asthma. Out door pollutants include diesel exhaust particles, which have recently been shown to have epigenetic effects during early life (Chapter 8). Indoor pollutants (other than cigarette smoke) that have been linked with asthma or allergy include formaldehyde (in new housing or buildings with extensive wooden surfaces),[40] home gas appliances[41] and cooling systems.[42] Although we have recommended that parents minimise exposure to indoor air pollutants,[43] we have also noted that this is not based on strong evidence, and more studies are needed to provide more specific recommendations.

6. *Allergy vaccinations?* An early 'vaccination' could be an ideal solution for preventing allergic disease, but an effective way of achieving this is still a fair way off. The closest thing we have like this now is 'immunotherapy' (Chapter 10), which is currently only recommended as treatment for established allergy (rather than prevention). This involves deliberate but gradual and controlled exposure to allergens (either by

injection or under the tongue) with a view to retraining the immune response. Clearly this is only directed at an allergen that someone is already allergic to (such as bee venom or house dust mites). There is some evidence that children already on immunotherapy for one allergy (house dust mite) are less likely to develop new allergies.[44] It is much harder to imagine how this technology could be applied more generally to 'prevent' allergic responses to a whole range of allergens that diverse groups of young infants might potentially become allergic to. There have been some initial attempts to take a preventive approach by choosing a mixture of the most common inhaled allergens in young infants at risk of asthma. However, progress in this area is likely to be slow because of the important and necessary rigorous safety requirements that must be addressed in clinical trials involving 'immune interventions' in very young, otherwise well, children. While there is great potential in this area, these is also understandably great caution because we need to know more about the developing immune system before we implement these kinds of interventions.

WHERE DOES THIS LEAVE US?

Prevention should still be our ultimate goal. Although progress may seem frustratingly slow, we must remember that it is not that long since allergic disease became recognised as a significant health issue. We now have a much better understanding of the complexity of these conditions and their role in the broader story of immune disease. It is no longer feasible to anticipate simple solutions that will work for everyone. We understand the ultimate need to identify an individual's susceptibility to allergy (along with other diseases) and the most likely gene-environment interactions that could lead to disease in that person. From there we may be able to design more personalised strategies, tailoring what we *can* control in the environment to prevent many diseases. At the same time, we must be careful to do no harm and avoid unintended adverse consequences. Although there are yet many, many pieces in this puzzle, every new piece of research adds to this ever-expanding mosaic. Recent strides in technology are bringing these still futuristic ideas ever closer. None of this can be achieved without ongoing research.

10

Allergy in practice:
general principles of diagnosis and management

Here the secret processes of the medical mind are revealed! Well, they are not really so mysterious, but might provide a useful insight into what might pass through the mind of your physician during a consultation. It is really a matter of gathering clues and making deductions, usually based on the story and the physical evidence. In some cases we might want to call in the laboratory to look a little further. Many believe that we have come to rely too much on the modern laboratory and not enough on the deductive powers of our ancient art. When we have everything lined up, we sift the evidence, fix on the most likely scenario and see if we can exclude other suspects. Then we make a plan. This is based on the problem and the best solution, weighing up the pros and cons of any action. First do no harm. The cardinal rule. And of course the patient and/or the care-giver must be fully engaged whenever possible. Involved in the discussion. Involved in the decision. Committed to the plan. And have the capacity to follow through. Without this, success is much less likely.

· · ·

So, while we continue to dream about effective prevention, the reality of modern medicine is still focused on diagnosing and treating disease. Most medical training is therefore focused on recognising the signs and symptoms of a disease so we can identify it correctly and recommend the best treatment. Every medical student is taught that the essential steps in making a correct diagnosis are 1) taking a good history of the patient's 'symptoms', 2) making a thorough physical examination for 'signs' of disease and 3) proposing any relevant investigations or 'tests' that might confirm the diagnosis.

The first and most important step in making the correct diagnosis is taking a good history about the presenting complaint or symptom. Allergic disease is no exception. In fact we can usually get a very good idea of what is going on based on only what patients (or their parents) tells us. The history of allergy in immediate family members is also helpful in determining the likelihood of an allergic cause. A good physical examination can add more information and confirm suspicions, if there are any current signs of disease. In some allergic patients, the examination can be normal if they are not actually having an allergic reaction at the time. Others may have signs of asthma, eczema or rhinitis. Finally, and only after these initial steps, do we consider any diagnostic 'tests'. As with many other conditions, the tests must be guided by what we have learnt from the history and examination. This helps us choose the most appropriate tests and also helps us interpret them. Allergy tests in the absence of this vital background information about the patient's exact symptom history can be fairly meaningless. For example, we see many patients that have positive allergy tests to foods they eat without symptoms. With that history we can confidently advise them to keep eating. But for another patient with the same test result and a history of anaphylaxis, we are very careful to advise strict avoidance. This is why it is important to ask so many questions.

EARLY SYMPTOMS THAT SUGGEST ALLERGY

Symptoms of allergy can begin at any age, but this tendency often first appears in early childhood. The patterns of disease vary with age, although there are always exceptions. Food allergy and eczema are generally the first signs of allergic disease, often appearing within the first weeks or months of life. Symptoms of food allergy can range from skin rashes through to life threatening anaphylactic reactions (Chapter 11). Eczema is generally noted as a more chronic and recurring red, scaly, itchy rash that can occur on almost any part of the body in infants (Chapter 12). Children with these conditions are also at greater risk of developing other allergic diseases as they get older, including asthma and allergic rhinitis. Although asthma (allergic inflammation of the lower airways) may begin in the first years of life, it can be hard to diagnose at this age because symptoms of coughing, wheezing and shortness of breath (Chapter 13) are also common in young children with viral illnesses who don't have asthma. Similarly, symptoms of allergic rhinitis (allergic inflammation of the upper airways) such as nasal congestion, blockage and sneezing (Chapter 14) can also be nonspecific in young children. Allergy becomes a more likely cause when these symptoms are unrelated to infections. This natural progression from food related allergies to respiratory allergies is sometimes referred to as the 'Allergic March'. It is a useful model and a good rule of thumb, but on an individual basis many people do not strictly follow the 'model'. The chance of progression to 'respiratory' allergies is greatest in children with more severe eczema and food allergies. But many children do not progress from one disease to another, and some present only with asthma or allergic rhinitis without any previous history of eczema or food allergy. Sometimes the first symptoms of allergy may not appear until adulthood. All this underscores the high degree of variability in these conditions.

WHAT WE WANT TO KNOW IN THE ALLERGY HISTORY

The main objective when taking any patient history is an accurate idea of the type of symptoms, exactly how and when these began, and the pattern that they have shown since. The severity of symptoms is also very important as this will dictate the treatment approach needed. All these features will vary with each condition and with each patient. When allergy is suspected, we also aim to identify possible triggers. That means questions about the diet and the general environment that may make the symptoms worse. We also ask more general health questions about other related or unrelated conditions that can affect our diagnosis or the treatment options. Some patients have already tried certain treatments and it is useful to know if these were effective or not. A family history of allergies is important as it increases the probability that we are dealing with an allergic problem, and can be particularly useful in very young infants when the diagnosis of allergic conditions (such as asthma) can be more difficult. By the end of the history taking, we usually have a good idea of what we are dealing with and a clear direction for our subsequent examination and investigations.

WHAT WE LOOK FOR IN THE PHYSICAL EXAMINATION

The main purpose of any physical examination is to gather more clues that indicate the most likely diagnosis, the severity of the condition, and any associated problems. Usually there is a focus on the problem at hand, but many doctors take this opportunity to look for signs of any other conditions that might affect the health of the patient. We start very generally and then focus on particular areas. Our observations in fact start well before the actual examination. During the history taking we are often observing general appearance and wellness. Some patients, even little children, can have facial tell-tale signs of allergy such as skin creases and dark rings under the eyes, puffiness, mouth breathing or a crease along the end of their nose from repeated rubbing. We describe this appearance as 'allergic facies'. There may also be visible skin rashes that suggest eczema or other allergies. We then look at other general factors such as weight and growth, particularly in children who might be on restriction diets for suspected food allergies. The general appearance can also give important clues to general nutrition and any signs of deficiencies. If we see anything suspicious or out of the ordinary we look in more detail, otherwise we concentrate on the obvious areas that are suggested in the allergy history, such as the skin, nose, throat, chest and abdomen.

We look at the skin for signs of eczema, noting the distribution and severity (Chapter 12). Looking in the nose we can see if there is obstruction, swelling and secretions. We might apply pressure on the sinuses (either side of the nose and the forehead) to see if they are tender. Looking in the throat we can see the size of the tonsils, which can give a clue to whether the adenoid (nose tonsil) might also be swollen and contributing to obstructed breathing.

A blocked nose can mean blocked ears. That is because there is a drainage tube from the middle ear space (between the inner and the outer ear drum) into the nose. That is how we equalise the pressure when our ears 'pop'. If there is a lot of swelling in the nose, the tube can get blocked and the pressure drops and fails to equalise as air is resorbed. When the pressure drops, fluid can be drawn out from the tissues causing 'glue ear' which can affect hearing. This is a particular problem in young children, and the reason that we look to see if the ear drums are retracted ('sucked in') with a fluid level visible behind them. We might feel the glands in the neck, as these can be swollen if they are draining an infection in the throat, ears or sinuses.

Before we listen to the chest with our stethoscope, we look for chest deformities that can occur in longstanding asthma. If asthma is not well treated and patients have chronic extra work of breathing, this can cause a change in chest shape with a depression in the lower rib cage. This can be a clue about the disease severity and the disease control, even if there are no actual symptoms at the time. We might ask the patient to cough and listen to the sound of the cough, which can also give clues. An asthma cough is more 'dry and tight' compared to the 'loose' productive cough of bronchitis infections, or the 'barking seal' cough of croup. If a patient has symptoms of asthma at the time of examination, the chest may appear fuller than usual (or 'hyper-inflated') with extra effort of breathing, seen as in-drawing of the soft tissue between the ribs and at the base of the neck. If wheezing is obvious, we may be able to hear it even without the stethoscope. This is a noisy whistling sound usually worse when the patient exhales, because the small air tubes in the chest are narrowed (Chapter 13).

The rest of the examination will depend on what we have found so far. But by the time we have finished our history and examination, we have sometimes already made a diagnosis or should have enough information to formulate a plan for further investigations.

TESTING FOR ALLERGIC ANTIBODIES

Allergy tests are typically used to confirm a suspected allergy, but in some cases they are also used to exclude an allergy and show that it is safe to be exposed to a particular allergen. Although there are many potential allergens we can test for, it is important that we select a 'short list' based on the history. The history is also important in determining the significance of the result. It is pointless and unnecessary to test randomly for allergies. This is because not all people with positive tests have symptoms, and not all people with symptoms have a positive test.

There are two main methods for detecting specific allergies, either a blood test or an allergen skin prick test (SPT). Both of these tests measure allergic (IgE) antibodies (Chapter 3) to specific allergens, such as foods, pollens, dust mites and insect venom. Positive tests only confirm the presence of the antibodies, they do not necessarily indicate whether a patient will actually have symptoms, what kind of symptoms might occur or how severe those symptoms might be. On the other hand, a negative allergy test means that an IgE-mediated reaction to that allergen is very unlikely.

The allergen-skin prick test (SPT)

This is the quickest and the cheapest test to do. It is also generally more sensitive (better at detecting positive tests) than the blood test and the patients have the result immediately. The main limitation is that it needs to be done by trained staff and is therefore mainly used in a specialist setting. It involves placing suspected allergens on the skin (usually on the forearm or the back) and superficially pricking the skin so that the allergen can come in contact with immune cells in the skin. If patients have specific IgE to a particular allergen on their cells (mast cells), the allergen will bind and cross-link the IgE molecules on the cell surface and cause the cells to release histamine (Chapter 3). This causes a small itchy lump (wheal) to appear usually within 15–20 minutes. The size of the wheal is measured as an indication of the level of antibodies. If there are no IgE antibodies nothing happens, and the test is considered negative. Another advantage of this test is that it can be used to test a much wider range of allergens than are available on blood tests. For example, we can test for allergy to almost any fresh food by applying a small droplet directly to the skin. The SPT is very safe, but clearly involves exposing patients to a tiny amount of allergens that they might be highly allergic to. In practice, a small droplet containing allergen rarely causes more than local irritation, even in patients with a history of anaphylaxis. But this extremely small risk is another reason that SPT is generally only used by trained staff. Because this test relies on the release of histamine from the patient's own cells, the test will not work properly if a patient has been on antihistamines. This is why we often ask patients not to have antihistamines (if possible) in the week prior to their appointment. Medications that have antihistamine-like properties, such as antidepressants can also interfere with the allergy SPT. Other medications that allergic patients may be taking (such as steroids) do not interfere with this test.

The allergy blood test

IgE antibodies to specific allergens can also be detected in the blood. This is a standardised laboratory test that can easily be requested by non-specialists as well. It is sometimes still referred to as a 'RAST' based on the name of a laboratory method (radioallergosorbent testing) used to detect the specific IgE to each individual allergen, although many laboratories use newer methods these days. This test is more expensive and unlike the SPT the results are not available during the consultation. While most laboratories offer a comprehensive range of allergen tests, this is still more limited compared to what can be done by SPT. One advantage over the SPT is that it can still be validly performed in patients who have taken antihistamine medications. This test usually provides an actual level of IgE antibody detected in the serum that is specific for each allergen tested. When the levels are below the detection limit of the assay (too low to detect) the test is deemed 'negative'. The level of total IgE can also be measured, but this is less useful. High levels often suggest allergy, but don't indicate what the antibodies are directed towards, and can also be elevated in patients with parasitic infections or other non-allergic immune disorders.

INTERPRETING THE ALLERGY TESTS: THE IMPORTANT DISTINCTION BETWEEN 'ATOPY' AND ALLERGIC DISEASE

When the allergy tests (SPT or RAST) are positive this confirms only that the patient is 'sensitised' to the allergen. 'Atopy' is the term often used to describe this tendency to produce specific IgE antibodies after exposure to common environmental allergens.

But this does not mean that they will have any signs or symptoms of disease. While many patients with allergic diseases are 'atopic', some are not, and, conversely, some patients with atopy do not manifest atopic disease.

USING THESE IgE ALLERGY TESTS FOR DIAGNOSIS, MONITORING AND TREATMENT DECISIONS

Allergy tests are initially used to confirm (or exclude) an allergy. After that they can be used to monitor how allergies are developing or changing with age, especially in children. They can provide evidence, much hoped for, that a child is outgrowing their food allergy, and it is time to consider a food challenge (Chapters 1 and 11). For a limited number of common foods, researchers have defined specific IgE levels that can be used as a guide to predicting the likelihood of a reaction during a food challenge. Either way, this is a slow process, and there is no need to repeat these tests too often. In our clinic, we rarely do these tests more than once a year in young children, and much less frequently as they get older. Once our patients reach their teens and their allergy patterns are more set, we may not repeat the allergy tests at all, unless something changes in their clinical history.

ALLERGEN 'CHALLENGES': THE DEFINITIVE TEST OF ALLERGIC REACTIONS

The most conclusive way to demonstrate or exclude an allergy is to see what happens when the patient is directly exposed under controlled, supervised medical conditions. This is called an allergen 'challenge' and should only be considered when the possible benefits outweigh the risks. Again this can be used to confirm or exclude a diagnosis, or to try to confirm development of immune tolerance when there are signs (i.e. on the IgE tests) that the allergy maybe resolving. When there is a history of recent, convincing and severe reactions (such as a clear anaphylactic reaction to a bee sting or eating peanut) it is difficult to justify a challenge. The method of challenge varies with the allergens tested. 'Food challenges' involve eating the allergenic food, starting with very small amounts and building up to a typical 'serving' size over a few hours. This is usually done according to strict protocols with each 'dose' carefully measured. It is graded so that patients can be observed closely after each increment. The challenge is usually terminated early if the patient develops significant symptoms. 'Nasal provocation challenges' and 'bronchial inhalation challenges' can be used to confirm responses to inhaled allergens, but these are not routine. 'Drug challenges' are used to assess possible drug reactions, most commonly to antibiotics (Chapter 15). Again, these are used mainly where the history is unclear and the probability of a severe reaction is low (based on IgE tests if these are available). Once again, if the history is convincing and the reaction severe then it is safer to just avoid that drug in future and use an alternative. In the past, insect 'venom challenges' (i.e. bee venom injections) were done in some centres after the completion of immunotherapy to confirm that patients were no longer reactive, but this is rarely done these days.

All of these procedures involve potential risk of anaphylaxis, and should only be performed in a specialised medical setting by well-trained staff. It is important that the patients and/or caregivers understand the reason for the procedure and give informed consent. Most centres require written consent before proceeding. In all cases, appropriate emergency facilities and treatments (such as adrenaline) must be immediately available.

GENERAL PRINCIPLES IN MANAGING ALLERGIC DISEASE
After making the correct diagnosis, there are a few general principles that we can apply to most situations. Above all, it is important to educate the patients and/or their parents during every step of this process.

Firstly, if we have identified a trigger, the first step is to avoid it. If allergens were the only trigger and could be completely avoided, then treatment would be simple. In reality, avoidance can be difficult and not always possible. Meticulous avoidance is most critical in situations where exposure can be life threatening, such as food anaphylaxis. This is time-consuming and stressful and even then accidental exposures are not uncommon. Complete avoidance of inhaled allergens such as dust mites, which can trigger asthma and rhinitis, is virtually impossible for people living in endemic regions. Some reduction in levels is usually the best we can hope for. Grass pollens, carried for long distances in the wind, are even more difficult to avoid. This aspect of the treatment plan is focusing on preventing an episode, and there may be other factors (apart from allergens) that can also be avoided, such as cigarette smoke in asthma, or skin irritants in eczema.

Secondly, we propose a clear treatment plan to follow when symptoms are triggered. This is usually an immediate response strategy for acute symptoms, which will vary according to the condition. Having well prepared emergency 'action plans' is especially important for potentially life threatening conditions such as severe asthma and anaphylaxis. This requires that patients and/or their caregivers are familiar with the medications needed, as well as when and how these should be given. It is critical that they also know at what point they should call for expert help.

The third aspect of management is the longer-term control of the disease. Asthma, rhinitis and eczema can be more chronic in some patients and regular medications can help control symptoms and reduce the risk of acute flares (Chapters 11–13). These treatments are also directed at controlling symptoms of the allergic disease rather than curing the underlying allergy. Again, this depends on the condition and severity.

Finally, in some patients we consider more definitive modification of the underlying immune response using immunotherapy.

This is used on a selective basis depending on the kind of disease, the severity and the response to other treatment.

IMMUNOTHERAPY: A 'CURATIVE' STRATEGY TO REVERSE THE ALLERGIC RESPONSE

Immunotherapy is currently the only established method of altering the 'natural history' of allergic disease. It surprises many patients to learn that immunotherapy has been in use for more than one hundred years (it recently celebrated its centennial),[1] long before IgE was even discovered and long before we knew much about allergic disease at all. Even now we are still uncovering the underlying mechanisms.

Immunotherapy is used in a range of allergic conditions; most commonly for allergic rhinitis, asthma and stinging insect allergy. There is growing evidence that some patients with eczema who are receiving immunotherapy for these other conditions (i.e. house dust mite immunotherapy for allergic rhinitis) also experience improvement in their skin disease. In all of these situations the objective is to induce lasting immune tolerance to the allergen in question, so that exposure no longer induces symptoms. Oral immunotherapy (OIT) for food allergy is very dangerous and still experimental because of the significant safety concerns, but there is hope that standardised protocols could eventually be optimised for clinical practice (Chapter 11).

While there are a number of methods and dosing regimes available, all immunotherapy protocols involve gradually giving increasing doses of allergen over an extended period, beginning at extremely low levels. Even though patients may be highly allergic, this graded exposure during the 'induction phase' minimises serious side-effects. Once patients reach a full dose, they enter the 'maintenance' phase which involves continued regular allergen exposure for a longer period (sometimes up to 3–5 years depending on the protocol and the method used). There is very strong evidence for the effectiveness of immunotherapy; however, this depends on the patients' history as not all are likely to benefit. To maximise the effectiveness and minimise the risks, it is very important to follow the prescribed protocol.

Although patients can be quite quickly 'desensitised' (rendered temporarily unresponsive to allergen) this may not be lasting unless there is continued long-term exposure. A more 'permanent' tolerance is driven by changes in underlying cellular immune function, with induction of regulatory T cells (Chapter 5) and suppression of the Type 2 allergic T cell response (Chapter 5). This is a more gradual process and is the reason for the extended maintenance phase of therapy. But curiously enough, IgE allergy tests often remain positive even after immunotherapy has successfully suppressed cellular reactions to allergens. The reasons for this are not fully understood, but there is some evidence that therapy induces IgG 'anti-allergic' antibodies that inhibit the effects of the IgE allergic antibodies (Chapter 3). For this reason, it is not useful to track the response to immunotherapy by measuring specific IgE levels.

Traditionally, immunotherapy has been given by subcutaneous injection (SIT), typically in the upper arm much like a vaccine. Regular injections can be a psychological barrier for many patients, especially children. In more recent years an oral method has been developed, giving the allergen under the tongue (or 'sublingually') as drops or dissolving tablets. The use of sublingual immunotherapy (SLIT) is increasing with more and more evidence of its effectiveness. It has generally been more expensive and it is still not available in many regions.

The decision to use immunotherapy is based on weighing up the 'burden of disease' against the 'burden of the treatment'. Clearly, in patients with mild disease who respond well to other treatment, this course of therapy is hard to justify. Immunotherapy to a specific allergen should only be used when the patient has proven sensitisation to that allergen, with evidence that the allergen is a significant contributor to symptoms. The best candidates for immunotherapy are those who experience a significant burden of disease, with limited response to their other treatments and who are sensitised to only a few allergens. When patients are allergic to a large number of allergens, immunotherapy may be less effective. However, even these patients can experience some benefit.

There are risks involved in immunotherapy. We are giving allergen to allergic patients, so it is important that precautions are taken. Most side effects are mild, and many patients will experience redness and swelling around the injection site. This can be reduced by taking antihistamines a few hours before the injection. More extensive, but still moderate reactions such as rhinitis, mild asthma, or hives are less common and estimated to only occur in one in 1500 injections.[2] More severe reactions are rare, but patients should always be made aware of the risk of life threatening anaphylaxis which has been said to occur about once per million injections.[3] Protocols are designed to minimise these risks and precautions should always be in place, but it is a further reason that therapy should be reserved for patients where the burden of disease justifies the risk. All patients should be observed for at least thirty minutes (and preferably forty-five minutes) after each injection even when they are on their maintenance doses. This allows immediate access to medical treatment if reaction occurs.[4] An important exception to using immunotherapy is in patients with very severe, unstable asthma. In these patients it is often not recommended because the risk of the immunotherapy injections tipping them into a severe asthma attack is considered too great.

For all these reasons, immunotherapy is a significant under-taking. Patients need to be fully informed and prepared to make the commitment. It is not for the faint hearted. But for those who respond there are clear benefits, with reductions in symptoms, better control of disease and complete resolution in some cases.

For conditions such as bee venom allergy (Chapter 15), immunotherapy is usually curative. In this condition the benefits far outweigh the risk and immunotherapy should be recommended for all patients who have had significant systemic reactions. There are also clear benefits in allergic rhinitis and asthma, and some emerging evidence that early treatment can prevent the development of new allergic diseases[5] and new sensitisations.[6] Further research into preventative immunotherapy (Chapter 9) is therefore a future goal.

THE PROGNOSIS AND 'NATURAL HISTORY' OF ALLERGIC DISEASES

It is useful to be able to give patients and/or their parents a rough guide to what the future might hold. Conditions such as food allergies, eczema, asthma and rhinitis tend to follow age-related patterns (discussed respectively for each condition in Chapters 11–14). Some conditions typically resolve spontaneously, some are more likely to persist without interventions such as immunotherapy. Clearly, if disease is mild and likely to resolve naturally with age, it is harder to justify these more demanding long-term therapies. Every patient follows their own individual course, but the general trends can be useful, particularly when weighing up treatment decisions. So there are always individualised choices that need to be made for each patient, and each allergic condition is different. But there are some general principles that apply in the diagnosis and management of each specific allergic condition, and the chapters that follow go on to discuss the basic approach to each of the common allergic diseases.

11

Food allergy – the new allergy epidemic

The vast majority of new referrals to our clinic are now for potentially serious food allergies. We face the same problems as nearly everyone else: too many new patients, not enough trained staff and not even enough clinic rooms to see the patients. Because food allergy is such a recent and growing problem, health care systems around the globe have simply not had time to catch up. It is now estimated that 220–520 million people may suffer from food allergy globally.[1] It takes time to train specialists. And resources. It also takes time and, unfortunately, avoidable deaths, to convince governments to put more funding towards training in anaphylaxis and allergy and towards specific allergy healthcare services. This is an international problem. And finding solutions requires an international effort. But the implementation of services often remains at the mercy of local funding and local governments, and that brings local challenges. International expert bodies, such as the World Allergy Organization (WAO), are playing a key role in addressing this problem at every level through promoting awareness, education and research into common allergic conditions, including food allergy.[2]

While we were feeling confident that asthma had reached a peak in the industrialised countries, this new epidemic of food allergy has been sneaking up on us. It is quite incredible how common this has become. It is also still quite puzzling why this surge in food allergy has lagged so far behind the epidemic of asthma and other allergies. Are the same environmental changes responsible? Is this just a sign of earlier and more significant effects? Or is something else happening now? This problem has only surfaced quite recently and we don't have the answers yet. More research is the only way that we will be able to answer these questions and solve this growing problem.

• • •

Food allergy is a serious and growing burden for many communities. There has been limited awareness and persistent skepticism about its significance, even amongst medical practitioners. This may be because the rise in this allergy has only been quite recent. But now with pre-schoolers showing a five-fold rise in serious food reactions over just the last ten years, there is an urgent need for action and awareness.[3] Many countries are now addressing this with food allergy and anaphylaxis awareness programs in both professional and community settings. Sadly, awareness is often driven by the reports of avoidable deaths from anaphylactic food allergy. But these high-profile cases have drawn attention to the much larger and growing number of people dealing with the pressure and anxieties of food allergy every day. This potentially life threatening condition is a very real and growing problem.

WHAT IS FOOD ALLERGY?

Food allergies are abnormal immune reactions to foods. The most critical part of this definition is in the 'immune' nature of the reaction, which makes food allergy quite distinct from non-immune reactions such as lactose intolerance, food poisoning or chemical reactions, which are often mislabeled as food allergies. Lactose intolerance is perhaps the most common reaction that is incorrectly labeled as food allergy (discussed later in this Chapter). It is due to a reduced ability to digest the lactose (sugar) in milk and is quite different from milk allergy, which is an immune reaction to the 'protein' in milk.

There are several different kinds of immune reaction that can occur to foods and these have been broadly divided into 'IgE-mediated' food allergy and '*non*-IgE mediated' food allergy.

IgE-mediated food allergy, as the name suggests, is caused by the allergic IgE antibodies to foods. It is the most common kind of food allergy, and also the best characterised. The symptoms occur rapidly, within less than an hour (often within minutes) of food exposure. This makes the diagnosis usually fairly obvious from the history and when IgE allergy tests such as the SPT and RAST (Chapter 10) are usually positive.

Non-IgE mediated food allergy is more difficult to diagnose because the symptoms can be delayed for hours or even days after the food exposure, and because the IgE tests are negative. These conditions are less common, but probably also underestimated because they are harder to recognise. In most cases the only clear way to diagnose these conditions is food elimination (to see if symptoms improve) followed by a formal food challenge (to see if symptoms recur). Part of the reason for the lack of a clear laboratory test is because this is a 'mixed bag' of conditions and because the underlying immune mechanisms are not understood. In general, these conditions are believed to be caused by abnormal T cell responses. A range of gastrointestinal syndromes fall under this banner, and some children with eczema also have non-IgE mediated food-induced symptoms.

How common is food allergy?

Food allergy is most common in young children but, because of the rapidly rising rates of food allergy, it is difficult to get accurate figures of the current prevalence. Although it was previously estimated that around 6 per cent of children under three years of age have food allergies,[4] this is likely to significantly underestimate current rates. Newer data from high prevalence areas like Australia suggest at least double that rate now. A recent Melbourne study found that over 20 per cent of infants were sensitised to foods after performing allergy skin prick tests (SPT) on almost 5,000 one year olds attending community health clinics. Around half of these children had clinical reactions when challenged with the food.[5] This is consistent with the staggering increase in hospital admissions for anaphylaxis in preschool children.[6] There is also evidence that specific food allergies, such as peanut, have risen dramatically.[7] These observations provide convincing evidence that food allergy rates are continuing to rise and that this is an important and significant public health issue.

FOODS MOST COMMONLY IMPLICATED IN FOOD ALLERGY

Although any food can potentially evoke an allergic reaction, in practice we see that over 90 per cent of childhood food allergies in are caused by hen's egg, cow's milk, soy, peanuts, tree nuts, wheat, fish and shellfish.[8] Some of these food allergies are typically transient, with tolerance developing by school age (for cow's milk, egg, soy and wheat), whereas others are more persistent and typically life-long (peanuts, tree nuts, and shellfish). The reason for these distinctly different age-related patterns is not clear.

SYMPTOMS THAT SUGGEST FOOD ALLERGY

Immediate reactions to foods are quite obvious, and usually due to allergic IgE antibodies to the food (i.e. 'IgE-mediated'). Symptoms can range widely from mild rashes to life threatening reactions and even death. Redness and swelling, typically of the lips and eyes, can be striking but are not always present. Itchy rashes are common and can be localised to areas where there has been direct food contact or more generalised to areas where there has been no clear contact. The typical allergy rash is due to histamine release and appears as raised pale welts surrounded by redness; often referred to as hives (or urticaria). These lesions vary widely in size and usually fade within hours. More serious symptoms occur when swelling affects the throat and makes breathing difficult. This is obvious when there is choking and noise breathing (called 'stridor'), but more subtle signs include hoarseness of the voice and coughing. It is important to look for these in young children who cannot explain that they have a tight feeling in their throat. Any of these 'airway' symptoms suggest a serious anaphylaxic reaction which can be life threatening. Massive histamine release can also cause a dangerous drop in blood pressure during anaphylaxis. Patients may appear pale and in extreme cases loose consciousness. This is very serious and can be fatal. Although most IgE-mediated reactions develop very quickly (usually within an hour and typically within minutes), symptoms can be delayed, although this is much less common. A milder, more localised form of IgE food allergy called 'oral allergy syndrome' occurs in older children and adults, who experience itching in and around their mouths after eating certain foods.

Vomiting after food ingestion can also be a symptom of many kinds of food allergy. This can occur as part of IgE-mediated reactions, usually soon after ingestion of the food. Vomiting and diarrhoea are also a feature of non-IgE gastrointestinal (gut) syndromes, when they may not occur until several hours after consuming the food. Poor weight gain or 'failure to thrive' can also occur in infants with non-IgE gastrointestinal food allergies due to inflammation in the gut. Nutritional problems can be a risk in food allergies that require multiple food avoidance, and they are the reason that dietary guidance is important in such cases.

Eczema can also be triggered by foods, but usually *only* in a subset of young children (Chapter 12). A flare of eczema can occur after an acute IgE-mediated reaction. Eczema can also be part of non-IgE mediated reaction with a delay of more than twenty-four hours before the exacerbation.

In a less common form of food allergy, the IgE reaction only occurs when the patient exercises after eating the particular food (called 'exercise-induced food anaphylaxis', see Chapter 15). It may take longer to diagnose this because symptoms only occur when eating of the food is followed by exercise (not by the food by itself or by exercise alone).

Another very rare and unusual form of food allergy is the 'Heiner syndrome' which occurs when food proteins (mostly cow's milk) induce a chronic inflammation in the lungs. This mainly occurs in infants and is very uncommon, but may be considered in a child fed cow's milk with unexplained difficulty in breathing and coughing blood possibly also with abdominal pain and blood in the faeces.

Then there are symptoms that can *sometimes* be related to food allergy. However, it is important to remember that *most* patients with these conditions do *not* have food allergy. This includes a small subset of infants with severe colic, persistent constipation and reflux, who show a *clear relationship* between food and symptoms. When there is no clear relationship, food allergy is very unlikely.

IgE-mediated food allergy in detail

This is the most common form of food allergy and generally appears in the first years of life when foods are first introduced, but can begin at any age. Reactions are typically 'immediate' occurring between several minutes and one–two hours after ingestion. They can be triggered by very small amounts of food allergen. Some patients develop reactions on minimal contact, and without actual ingestion. Breastfed infants can also react to foods their mothers have eaten although this is less common. This is thought to be due to traces of food proteins secreted into breast milk, and shows how sensitive IgE reactions can be.

Many parents report symptoms after the first apparent exposure to the food. However, IgE reactions generally mean there must be some pre-formed IgE 'memory' as a result of 'priming' following a previous exposure (Chapters 3 and 5). This indicates that the immune system must have been exposed previously, possibly through the placenta in pregnancy, possibly through the breast milk. There is even some suggestion that exposure through the skin can create sensitivity to food allergens before they are actually eaten (e.g. skin creams containing peanut oil).

As for all allergies, the general approach is to:
1. identify the triggering food(s)
2. avoid this/these while making sure that the nutritional needs are met
3. have a clear 'action plan' if there is an accidental exposure, and medical-alert bracelets to help emergency workers
4. educate the child, family, school and caregivers
5. monitor for possible resolution (and hope for progress with 'curative' interventions that are currently under research and development).

Education and support is a critical part of the management. With rising rates of anaphylaxis, many countries have developed national 'anaphylaxis action plans' to ensure a consistent standardised approach. An example, developed by the Australasian Society of Clinical Immunology and Allergy (ASCIA) is available at <www.allergy.org.au>.

Our medical students learn best from specific case studies, which illustrate the main issues. Here is a case that they presented to their colleagues for discussion in one of our case–base learning sessions.

IgE-MEDIATED FOOD ALLERGY

CASE STUDY

'Amy' is a 13 month old girl who was referred to our clinic by her family doctor following a reaction she had at her own birthday party four weeks earlier. She developed a bright red blotchy rash only a minute after eating only one bite of chocolate cake that contained egg, milk and peanuts. Amy's lips and eyes became severely swollen. Her mother, Tina, took her immediately to the family doctor who treated her with a non-sedating antihistamine. Amy was also pale, lethargic and wanted to go to sleep, but her rash and swelling gradually improved. She was almost 'back to normal' an hour later and was sent home with a referral to our allergy clinic.

A more detailed history in our clinic revealed that Amy had also had coughing, secretions and a hoarse cry during the reaction. As far as Tina was aware, Amy has never eaten egg or peanut before. However, Tina since remembered that Amy previously developed red marks on her hands after playing with egg cartons. She has been previously well apart from intermittent eczema from three months of age. Amy drinks cow's milk and dairy products with no apparent symptoms, or eczema flares. Tina had delayed Amy's twelve-month vaccinations because she had heard they might contain egg.

We performed allergy testing (SPT) which showed positive tests (a lump greater than 3 mm) against milk (5 mm), egg (10 mm) and peanut (4 mm). Amy's reaction was suspected to be due to egg, although a peanut reaction could not be excluded. We gave Amy her twelve month vaccinations and she had no reaction. Tina had anaphylaxis training and she was shown how and when to use the adrenaline injector that we prescribed in the event of any future reactions. She was also advised to avoid egg and peanut in Amy's diet. Tina was offered a dietician appointment to help her with this. Amy was booked for peanut challenge in hospital to determine the significance of the positive peanut test. This occurred a few months later and showed that Amy could eat peanuts without a reaction. She has been eating peanut butter two or three times a week since. She has continued having milk products because she has always tolerated these without symptoms. She has another appointment when she turns two for repeat SPT (and/or RAST) to egg. Tina has been advised that we will monitor the allergy tests anticipating *that, if these reduce with age, we will also proceed to an egg challenge hopefully to demonstrate that Amy is outgrowing her allergy.*

POINTS THIS CASE ILLUSTRATES

- IgE-mediated symptoms typically appear quickly (although they can be more delayed in some children)
- Amy had signs of anaphylaxis (hoarse voice and coughing) although this was not recognised at the time
- Lethargy and paleness can be signs of anaphylaxis in young infants
- Amy's symptoms of anaphylaxis should have been treated with adrenaline
- If patients have had a clear history of anaphylaxis, it is important that there is a clear 'action plan' for patient/carers to follow in the event of future reactions (including access to adrenaline)
- Antihistamines are useful for milder allergic reactions, but will not treat anaphylaxis
- If anti histamines are used, they should be a non-sedating variety to avoid masking drowsiness that can be a sign of anaphylaxis
- If a food is tolerated without symptoms, it should be continued in the diet even if the allergy tests is positive (such as milk in this case)
- When a patient has a positive test, but it is not known if they will have symptoms, a food challenge can be useful (as for peanut in this case where the test was positive). This must be done under medical supervision and is not done if the risk of reaction is deemed high (if the allergy test score is very high). For some common foods, cut-off levels have been generated to predict risk but these are only guides (based on probability rather than certainty) and these levels vary between centres and local practices. Many other factors need to be considered in the decision to perform a food challenge.
- Some vaccines are cultured in chicken embryos (such as the measles mumps and rubella 'MMR' vaccine), and may contain minuscule amounts of egg protein. Because the levels are so small these can be given safely to children with egg allergy. At present this is less

clear for the influenza vaccines. These are also derived from chicken embryos, but egg protein content can vary with different influenza vaccines. Although these vaccines can be given safely in most children with egg allergies (which is the practice in my centre), reactions have been reported and in some regions flu vaccinations are not recommended in these children. Because of international variations in recommendations (at the time of writing) it best that parents of egg allergic children discuss this with their specialist.

We can still be cautiously optimistic that Amy will out grow her egg allergy. In the past we have generally seen that allergies to egg, soy or dairy products typically improve and resolve by school age. While this is still true, there is some evidence that a growing proportion of these children are showing persistence of their allergies.[9]

Many children go through a period of 'partial' tolerance when they are able to tolerate well-cooked egg (in baked foods) before they are able to tolerate less cooked forms of egg (such as scrambled or soft-boiled eggs). This is because cooking partially destroys the egg allergen to a level where it can be tolerated by patients with mild to moderate egg allergy. We generally encourage these patients to eat well-cooked egg in the hope that regular exposure may accelerate 'complete' tolerance to all forms of egg, although this remains to be proven.

The prognosis of other IgE-mediated food allergies is more guarded, especially allergies to peanut, tree nut and shellfish, which are generally persistent. However, around 20 per cent of young children with peanut allergy appear to spontaneously outgrow their allergy, so it is still important to monitor these children for evidence of tolerance. This can be done by monitoring the specific IgE levels, but ultimately the only way to prove tolerance is by undertaking a food challenge.

Food challenges (as described in Chapter 10) are the definitive measure of allergy and when an allergy may be resolving. They are also useful when allergy test results are equivocal or the significance unclear. Food challenges are usually performed in hospital because of the risk of anaphylaxis. Where the risk of reaction is very high (a recent anaphylactic reaction or very strongly positive allergy tests) challenges are generally not done because they place a patient at unnecessary risk. However, when the risk of reaction is very low (a history of mild allergic reactions and a negative skin prick test) challenges can be done safely at home by parents. This is a critical decision that needs to be made in consultation with a specialist.

The greatest anxiety with food allergy is the risk of death from an accidental exposure. However, even though food allergies are most common in young children, deaths from anaphylaxis are very rare in preschool children. Deaths are more likely to occur in adolescents and adults, and even then these are very uncommon in well-managed patients. The chances are greater when appropriate precautions and emergency plans are not in place. Poorly controlled asthma is a particular risk factor for death, so we always stress the need for good asthma control in people with food allergy. This underscores the need for good education for patients/care-givers and the community at large.

A CURE FOR FOOD ALLERGY COULD NOW BE WITHIN REACH

The most promising development in this field is the prospect of curative therapy for persistent food allergies, known as both oral immunotherapy (OIT) and 'specific oral tolerance induction' (SOTI). The idea behind this, much like other immunotherapy (Chapter 10) is gradual incremental exposure to promote tolerance. This is not a new idea. In 1908 a physician named Dr Schofield published an interesting report in the noted medical journal, *Lancet*. He described a case of a thirteen year old boy who had what he labelled 'egg poisoning'.[10] He describes symptoms suspiciously similar to those of serious egg allergy. Food allergy was then so rare that it was not really recognised. Dr Schofield's remedy was to use pills that contained 1:10,000 raw egg, and to increase the boy's intake over eight months so that he was eventually eating whole eggs with no reaction. He successfully cured this boy's egg allergy. Food allergy was still rare and this insightful approach was in many ways ahead of its time.

Nearly one hundred years on and we are only just starting to revisit these ideas. There have been a series of more recent reports successfully using the same approach to 'cure' patients with anaphylactic reactions to egg, milk and peanuts.[11] As for other forms of immunotherapy there is a build-up (induction) phase and success then depends on regular exposure to the food allergen (during the maintenance phase, which continues for many months, and usually years). More recently, OIT has entered clinical trials to optimise protocols and to study the immune effects in more detail. Side effects are very common and there is a high risk of serious reactions especially during the build-up phase. It is also unclear how long the maintenance phase needs to be to achieve a 'permanent' immune tolerance, or even if this can be achieved in all patients. There are also reports of serious reactions (life threatening anaphylaxis) in patients who have had interruptions in their maintenance regime. Because of the serious consequences of this therapy, OIT remains a research tool at this time, while more studies are done to maximise the effectiveness and minimise the risks. There is growing anticipation for the day that OIT will be widely available in routine care. But this should be tempered by realistic expectations that this (OIT) may not be the answer for all patients. In the meantime, there are still many questions to be answered and we still ultimately aim for safer, more universally effective, treatments.

ECZEMA AND FOOD ALLERGY

There can be important links between eczema and food allergy, particularly in young children. However, not all children with eczema have food allergy and foods should only be avoided in cases where there is a clear relationship between the food and exacerbation of symptoms. This is discussed more fully in Chapter 12.

GASTROINTESTINAL FOOD ALLERGY SYNDROMES

A range of gastrointestinal syndromes can occur as a result of immune reactions to foods. These are generally *non*-IgE mediated reactions and appear to be due to poorly understood cellular reactions (although some patients can have 'mixed' IgE and non–IgE symptoms). The symptoms depend on which part of the gut is affected most, which can include oesophagus, the small intestine, the large intestine, or both. The main conditions are summarised here:

Name of condition (all induced by food protein)	Part of gut involved	Main symptoms
Eosinophilic oesophagitis ('EO' or 'EE' in North America)	Oesophagus (upper part of the gut that connects the mouth with the stomach)	Infants: vomiting and regurgitation, food refusal or aversion (in severe cases: irritability and poor weight gain) Older children and adults: difficulty swallowing, pain or indigestion
Enteropathy	Small intestine	Chronic diarrhoea, anal excoriation (redness and irritation), poor weight gain, nutritional deficiencies
'FPIES' (food protein induced enterocolitis syndrome)	Large and small intestine	Severe diarrhoea and vomiting (can be associated with severe circulatory collapse)
Proctocolitis	Lower large intestine (lower end of the colon and rectum)	Flecks of blood in the stools, but patients are rarely unwell

In general, the diagnosis is based on the clinical *history* of reaction because IgE allergy tests are usually *negative* and there are no other standard laboratory tests. Symptoms are usually delayed for several hours after ingestion; in some cases more than twenty-four hours later. Larger amounts of food are generally required to trigger these reactions (compared with IgE-mediated reactions). The best way to confirm the diagnosis is to eliminate the suspected food for a period of time to achieve improvement of symptoms and then to perform a deliberate re-challenge (reintroduction to demonstrate exacerbation of symptoms). If there is no improvement on withdrawal and/or no clear exacerbation on re-challenge, the food is unlikely to be implicated and further avoidance of that food is not justified. In practice, when there has been possible improvement after dietary elimination, parents/patients are often reluctant to re-challenge and undertake this final diagnostic step even when the symptoms were mild. These decisions should be made with medical consultation, especially if there is a history of severe symptoms, in which case the re-challenge is usually delayed until the risk is considered low.

The following cases illustrate these main gastrointestinal conditions:

EOSINOPHILIC OESOPHAGITIS

CASE STUDY

Sarah is a two year old girl who has a history of vomiting, regurgitation and food refusal. She is quite irritable after eating. This is starting to affect her weight gain. She also has a history of eczema and asthma. So does her mother. She has been seen by a gastroenterologist for suspected reflux and has not responded to the usual treatments. An endoscopy and biopsy of her oesophagus showed inflammation with high numbers of eosinophils, cells associated with allergy (Chapter 3), on microscopic examination. Allergy tests showed positive for allergy to house dust mite, but not to common foods. In consultation with an allergist and a dietician,

Sarah was placed on an elimination diet for the most common allergens (cow's milk, soy, egg, wheat, peanuts and tree nuts). There was partial improvement, and she was also placed on a trial of swallowed steroid aerosols (that she also inhales for her asthma). Her symptoms and a repeat biopsy both showed significant improvement. The plan is to eventually reintroduce the foods she is avoiding, one at a time, to see which cause an exacerbation of her symptoms. This will prevent unnecessary avoidance and allow a more focused elimination diet.

POINTS THIS CASE ILLUSTRATES

- This condition is often not recognised and patients can be mislabeled as having gastro-oesophageal reflux
- Patients with eosinophilic oesophagitis do not respond well to treatments for reflux
- The diagnosis needs to be made on a biopsy (endoscopy), which shows a classic appearance
- Patients may have other allergic disease (such as eczema and asthma) as in this case
- IgE tests to foods can be negative or positive (due to associated tendencies for IgE disease allergy), but this disease is not clearly IgE mediated
- There are several approaches to treatment including extensive elimination diets, or more selective elimination diets (as used here)
- Because there is allergic inflammation of the oesophagus, some patients respond to the anti-inflammatory effects of topical steroids. This is similar to using topical steroids on the skin in eczema. The best way of delivering the steroid to the surface of the oesophagus is swallowing the same steroids that are inhaled in asthma treatment. Patients use the same 'puffer device' but swallow rather than inhale. These swallowed aerosols are a much lower dose than steroid tablets and there is minimal absorption. This means there are very few side-effects
- Endoscopies are used to monitor progress.

The incidence of eosinophilic oesophagitis (EO) has risen significantly as part of the allergy epidemic, and many patients show other allergic tendencies. The diagnosis must be made by biopsy which requires an endoscopy under anaesthetic. While there is growing awareness of EO, it is probably still under-recognised because the diagnosis depends on a biopsy. EO can improve or persist with age. If it persists, the pattern of symptoms changes with age; from vomiting and regurgitation in young infants through to difficulty swallowing and indigestion in older children and adults. Specialists can use IgE allergy tests to guide the elimination diets, but offending foods may not return a positive IgE test. Some specialists use a different form of allergy skin test that can pick up 'cell-mediated' reactions. This is also known as a 'patch' test, and involved placing a food under an occlusive dressing for more than 48 hours to see if a local reaction develops. There is still debate over the usefulness of this test, and it is not available in many centres. Elimination diets can be very effective, but also very demanding and not very enjoyable in older children and adults. In young infants very elemental formulas (where the milk proteins are broken down to their amino acid building blocks) are used to provide nutrition without any allergens. In many counties these are not available without specialist prescription. Older patients often opt for selective elimination and swallowed steroid aerosols as a compromise that is easier to achieve. This decision is also influenced by the severity of symptoms. Periodic challenges are important to avoid or minimise unnecessary dietary restrictions.

FPIES (food protein induced enterocolitis syndrome)

CASE STUDY

Steven is a six month old boy who developed protracted vomiting and diarrhoea about three hours after his first feed with rice cereal mixed with cow's milk formula. Until then he had been fully breastfed. He became pale and floppy and was taken to the hospital where he was admitted and treated with antibiotics and intravenous fluids for dehydration and presumed infection. After two days he had fully recovered. All the tests for infection were negative and he was sent home. Two weeks later the baby sitter gave him a bottle of milk formula while his parents went out to dinner. The same symptoms recurred two hours later. He had to be rushed to hospital. This time a non-IgE mediated reaction to the cow's milk formula was suspected, because of the previous history. All allergy tests were negative. Milk and dairy products were excluded from his diet. He was given an observed test feed with rice cereal to make sure that this was not a trigger, and had no symptoms. His mother continued breastfeeding, but was advised to give a hypoallergenic (extensively hydrolysed) formula if complimentary milk feeds were necessary. She was also informed that Steven was highly likely to out-grow this condition, but that this could take several years.

POINTS THIS CASE ILLUSTRATES

- Steven has FPIES which is the abbreviation we often use for 'food protein induced enterocolitis syndrome'
- This non-IgE-mediated gastrointestinal syndrome can be serious
- It is usually only seen in young infants
- Symptoms can mimic other conditions such as serious infection (including meningitis and septicaemia) and may not be initially recognised as food allergy
- Symptoms are typically delayed for several hours after the feed, making the link with food less obvious
- There are no IgE-symptoms in these children, such as swelling and rashes (hives)
- Allergy tests are often negative
- The diagnosis of FPIES to cow's milk was made on the history (two episodes clearly related to cow's milk)
- Steven was given a test feed with rice to make sure that this was not

also a trigger (as rice is also a well-known food trigger in FPIES)

- Although extensively hydrolysed formulas (see later) are made from cow's milk, all the proteins have been broken down into small fragments that are more difficult for the immune system to 'see' as allergens.

This case illustrates a sometimes very dramatic and serious form of non-IgE food allergy. In some infants severe diarrhoea and vomiting can lead to serious circulatory collapse. The most common foods triggering FPIES are cow's milk and soy, although rice, wheat, oats and chicken are also known triggers, and infants may react to more than one food.[12] Infants with FPIES do not usually react to trace amounts of food. This may be why reactions to breast milk are uncommon, even when mothers are eating enough of the foods for traces of food protein to be present in their breast milk. FPIES almost always improves with age, but should be monitored by experts because of the risks associated with premature challenges; usually not done before two–three years of age.[13]

PROCTOCOLITIS

CASE STUDY

Heidi is very worried because her two month old baby girl, Jessica, has bright red flecks of blood in her stools. Jessica is a happy, thriving baby and does not seem distressed in any way. She is fully breastfed. Heidi enjoys dairy products, but was advised to avoid these in her own diet for a two week trial, while she continued to breastfeed. Jessica's bleeding settled within several days. Although this was very suggestive of cow's milk-induced proctocolitis, the paediatrician asked Heidi to start consuming milk and dairy products again to confirm the diagnosis. The symptoms recurred and Heidi returned to a dairy elimination diet for the duration of her breastfeeding. She was referred to a dietican to make sure that her calcium intake was supplemented with other foods and that her other nutritional requirements were satisfied.

POINTS THIS CASE ILLUSTRATES

- Jessica has food protein-induced proctocolitis, in this case induced by milk
- She is completely well otherwise and in no pain or distress. Although blood in the stool can look alarming, this in not serious. Only rare cases (with prolonged or severe bleeding) develop complications such as anaemia or poor weight gain
- Cow's milk is the most common trigger although soy, rice, and wheat are also implicated in some patients
- This can occur in breastfeeding infants (due to dairy proteins in the mother's diet) who are not actually ingesting the food directly.

Food protein-induced proctocolitis is due to allergic inflammation of the lower colon. Symptoms usually begin in the first three months of life and have often resolved by one year. It is another non-IgE condition. As in this case, symptoms can occur in breast-feeding infants, and a trial elimination of cow's milk products is useful. If symptoms do not improve, other foods (soy) can also be avoided. However, if there is still no improvement it may be necessary to cease breastfeeding and to place the infant on an extensively hydrolysed hypoallergenic formula.

PROTEIN-INDUCED ENTEROPATHY

CASE STUDY

Huey is a ten month old boy who has had persistent low-grade diarrhoea for several months. His bottom is red and excoriated (inflamed) and he is not gaining weight at the projected rate. He is unsettled and seems to be in pain. Because his symptoms seem to begin around the time he transitioned from breast milk to an infant formula (around six months of age), his mother Nancy suspected lactose intolerance. He showed some improvement when Nancy tried a lactose free formula, but this was only transient and the symptoms have continued despite also trying a soy formula. Although his symptoms began before he started wheat and gluten-containing cereals, Nancy was also worried about coeliac disease and excluded these foods while waiting to see the paediatrician. When he was assessed, Huey appeared malnourished with signs of anaemia and failure to thrive. Nancy was at her wit's end. The coeliac test was negative and the paediatrician started Huey on an extensively hydrolysed formula. Iron and folate supplements were also prescribed for his anaemia. His diarrhoea improved within the week and he became more settled. Over the following months Huey was monitored regularly and started to gain weight nicely. Nancy started gluten-containing foods without causing any exacerbations of his symptoms. She gradually introduced other foods to Huey's diet, but remains careful to avoid cow's milk and soy in his diet.

POINTS THIS CASE ILLUSTRATES

- Huey has a protein-induced enteropathy triggered by cow's milk and soy
- This mainly occurs in formula-fed infants
- Patients can be mislabelled as lactose intolerant. Lactose-free formula still contain intact cow's milk protein, which continues to trigger the inflammation that damages the gut lining. Removing lactose (a sugar) therefore only results in partial improvement and the underlying damage continues
- The signs and symptoms can be similar to coeliac disease, but are not triggered by gluten.

The inflammatory reaction in protein-induced enteropathy mainly occurs in the small bowel. This is where many nutrients are normally absorbed, so the chronic inflammation can lead to poor absorption and nutritional deficiencies. The signs and symptoms can be quite similar to coeliac disease, but coincide with the introduction of formula rather than gluten products. In severe cases an intestinal biopsy may be done to examine the bowel damage. Removing the offending food from the diet usually leads to a full recovery.

Lactose intolerance is often confused with food allergy. Lactose is a sugar in milk. When the lactose sugars are not digested properly they cause diarrhoea. This intolerance occurs when there is a deficiency or damage to the 'lactase' enzymes that are needed to digest lactose. These enzymes are located on the surface of the gut lining cells. If the gut lining is damaged (as occurs commonly but only temporarily after gastrointestinal infections) or more permanently (if there is a genetic deficiency) milk needs to be avoided to reduce the symptoms of lactose intolerance. Lactose intolerance can also occur as a secondary problem in protein-induced enteropathy, but it is not the cause. This is why there may be partial improvement when parents try a lactose-free formula. However, many parents do not realise that because lactose-free formula still contains normal cow's milk protein, it can continue to trigger symptoms and is not suitable in any kind of cow's milk allergy.

A LITTLE MORE ON INFANTS FORMULAS THAT ARE USED IN ALLERGIC DISEASE

This can be a confusing topic, even for health care workers, and it is worth some summary points, set out in the table below. Breast milk is almost always preferable to formula, except in rare instances where symptoms cannot be controlled by maternal elimination diets. When a cow's milk allergy is suspected the main alternatives to be considered are soy infant formula (depending on age and severity of allergy), extensively hydrolysed formula (eHF) or an amino acid formula (AAF).[14] Ideally, these formulas should only be continued if the allergy is subsequently confirmed and less allergenic formulas are not tolerated. There are regional variations in the preferential use of various formulas in the treatment of milk allergy, especially the use of soy formulas. AAF and eHF are expensive and not widely available in less affluent regions of the world. If patients with milk allergies tolerate a soy formula this is a reasonable alternative depending on the age of the child (below). It is not recommended in children under six months of age.[15] There are a number of formulas that are not suitable in milk allergy, and these include lactose-free cow's milk formula, partially hydrolysed formula, goat's milk formula (or other mammalian milks), A2 milk, rice milk, and oat milk.[16]

Formula	Description	Use
Standard infants formula	There are a huge range of formulas designed to mimic breast milk as closely as possible (many now with extra additives such as probiotics and PUFA). Most are derived from cow's milk (unless otherwise stated) and have intact cow's milk protein.	These are used as a standard breast milk substitute. Because these contain native cow's milk protein they must be avoided in cow's milk allergy.
Lactose-free infants formula	This is a cow's milk formula with the lactose sugar removed. It still contains intact cow's milk protein (which can cause allergic reactions).	In cases of lactose intolerance (which is not allergy). Should *not* be used in cow's milk allergy.
Partially hydrolysed formula (pHF)	This is a cow's milk formula with the protein partially broken down (into fragments called peptides). Some of the peptide fragments are still large enough to trigger an allergic reaction.	Allergy prevention (Chapter 9) where there is no evidence of milk allergy. These should *not* be used if infants develop a cow's milk allergy.

Formula	Description	Use
Soy formula	Soy formulas have modifications to better match infants' nutritional requirements (compared with standard soy milk). They usually do not contain cow's milk protein. Some children who are allergic to cow's milk are also allergic to soy. Experts recommend soy formula is not used until after six months of age.[17] As noted above, there are regional variations in the recommendations for soy.	Can be used as an alternative formula in many cow's milk allergic infants[18] (mainly after six months of age). If not tolerated, an eHF or AAF should be used.
Extensively hydrolysed formula (eHF)	This is a cow's milk formula with the protein extensively broken down into very small peptide fragments - this affects the taste, making eHF bitter compared to pHF and standard formulas. Most children with milk allergy can tolerate eHF.	Used for cow's milk allergy, particularly in those who are less than six months of age, or do not tolerate soy formula.
Amino acid formula (AAF)	AAF is also derived from cow's milk, where the proteins are completely broken down into amino acids, which are the basic building blocks of proteins. There are no milk peptides or proteins and this is the most hypoallergenic formula available. When these formulas are started early enough, infants don't seem to mind the bitter taste.	Used in cow's milk allergy, particularly severe allergies or when eHF and soy formula are not tolerated.

SOME OTHER SITUATIONS WHERE FOOD ALLERGY MAY BE
A FACTOR

In some young infants with gastro-oesophageal reflux disease (GORD), symptoms may be triggered by foods, particularly cow's milk protein. There are no features to distinguish these children, apart from the observations that symptoms usually begin within several days of starting milk protein in the diet. These children respond (i.e. with improved symptoms) to dietary elimination of cow's milk protein. To make the diagnosis, there should be strict avoidance for at least two to four weeks to demonstrate improvement, followed by re-challenge to confirm recurrence of symptoms.[18] Only then can continued exclusion be justified. If there is no change in symptoms, it is unlikely that the symptoms are due to cow's milk. As with other forms of cow's milk allergy, this also improves within the first one to two years of life.

There have been more controversial links between food allergy and other infant conditions such as colic and constipation in young infants. Most infants with these conditions *do not* have food allergy; however, a non–IgE mediated allergy may be suspected in a small subgroup of infants who show a relationship between the onset of symptoms and starting a formula. Infant colic (persistent irritability) usually only occurs in the first few months of life and usually resolves by four months. It is a poorly understood, multifactorial condition, but a subgroup of infants will respond to cow's milk elimination. This should be done with medical consultation. For formula fed infants this requires prescription of an eHF (or AAF) as a replacement formula (see table above). For breastfeeding infants, strict maternal elimination of cow's milk (all dairy) products can be considered for two to four weeks. If the milk protein is a factor, infants should generally show a response within a week.[19] Similarly, constipation in young infants which develops shortly after starting cow's milk in their diet, can be a sign of cow's milk allergy.[20] There is wide variation in normal bowel habits of young infants, and this is only relevant where the change in stool frequency and consistency coincides with starting a cow's milk formula (or another specific food). These infants can also respond to a trial of food elimination. In both conditions (infant colic and constipation) there are no diagnostic tests to distinguish infants who have cow's milk-induced symptoms from the majority of infants who do not. If there is no improvement with dietary elimination, continued restriction cannot be justified. As for other non-IgE conditions, when there is possible improvement, a rechallenge to the food is recommended to confirm the diagnosis (usually after four to six weeks). When symptoms are severe and do not respond to these measures, further medical consultation is important to exclude more serious underlying conditions.

• • •

We completely depend on proteins and many other nutrients for our survival. But these are all 'foreign' elements from our external environment and the immune system must learn quickly that they are not a threat. Most of these critical decisions need to be made in infancy, when the immune system is still immature. Food allergy is the result of an incorrect decision. The large variety of food allergy syndromes probably reflects the complexity of the immune system in the gut (Chapter 6). It is surprising in many ways that *most* of the time the immune system *does* get it right. But rising rates of food allergy clearly mean that changing environmental pressures are interfering with this important 'immune decision making' very early in development (Chapter 6).

12

Eczema and atopic dermatitis

Years later, and I am still getting Christmas cards from grateful parents of infants I have treated with eczema. This is another of the most rewarding aspects of our work. Just as the level of discomfort and distress of eczema can be extreme, so is the relief when it melts away with treatment. It is not hard to imagine the anxiety that parents face seeing their child covered with itchy, weeping sores. Agitated, scratching and bleeding into their bed sheets. So many sleepless nights. Stress. Exhaustion. We certainly can't cure this condition yet, but we can effectively control it in most patients until many of them outgrow it. This might not be a life-threatening condition, but the burden can be so great that the treatment can seem like a miracle. It is an ongoing battle, but once parents have seen a response, they are armed and ready for it next time. Having a plan of attack makes all the difference.

• • •

Eczema is one of the earliest signs of allergy. It can occur at any age, but often begins in the first months of life. As with other forms of allergic disease, there is convincing evidence that the incidence of eczema has increased,[1] now affecting at least 15–20 per cent of young children in western countries.[2] Although it is often dismissed as a trivial problem, eczema can be enormously distressing and can place significant strain on individuals and their families. Treatments can be time-consuming and potentially costly.

WHAT IS IT?

Eczema is a chronic and recurring inflammation of the skin. It is another complex disorder driven by both genetic and environmental factors. The contributing factors are likely to vary between individuals adding to evidence that, like asthma, eczema is not really a single condition. Although the underlying cause is not known, there is evidence that eczema is related to both an abnormal (leaky) skin barrier, as well as abnormal immune responses.

The terms and definitions used to describe this condition have changed over the years and can be confusing. The term 'dermatitis' really just means 'inflammation of the skin' and can have many other causes. The term 'atopic dermatitis' was intended to narrow this down to describe the eczema syndrome that is often (but not always) associated with IgE-mediated allergy. But although 'atopic dermatitis' is often used interchangeably with 'eczema', it is a less suitable term because the condition is not always 'atopic' (associated with IgE) and can be 'non-atopic' in 20–30 per cent of cases.[3] So I will stick with the term 'eczema'.

THE ROLE OF ALLERGY

Most patients (70–80 per cent) with eczema do have associated allergy,[4] with evidence of IgE-mediated sensitisations or signs of other allergic disease. In other words, they have atopic eczema. In very young infants the first clue to this might be a strong family history of allergies. Many of these children will go on to develop food allergy, asthma and rhinitis; particularly those children with more severe skin disease. Allergens can trigger the disease in allergic patients but there are usually many other triggers, and allergens are not the underlying cause of the condition. As already noted, around 20–30 per cent people with eczema have 'non-atopic eczema' without apparent IgE allergies. This suggests that although allergy is an important contributor, it is not essential for the development of eczema.

THE ROLE OF GENETICS AND OTHER FACTORS THAT INFLUENCE THE SKIN BARRIER

A subgroup of patients with eczema have a genetic variant in a gene called 'filaggrin', which is important for skin integrity. The result is more permeable skin. This has lead to growing speculation that more 'leaky' skin might be an initiating factor in the development of allergic disease. It has been proposed that defects in the skin barrier might increase the penetration of allergens to a point where they can come in contract with the local immune cells and initiate the allergic reaction.[5] In addition to genetic variations, a number of environmental factors can also disrupt the skin barrier to increase the permeability. These include bacteria (especially toxin-producing *staphylococcus* skin bacteria, or 'Staph'), allergens (like dust mites which produce chemical irritants), detergents and abrasive surfaces. Once an allergic reaction is initiated, more immune cells are recruited into the skin to produce many more inflammatory products, and this too contributes to the breakdown in skin barrier integrity. A vicious circle sets in and it is hard to work out what happened first. As with all complex genetic-environmental interactions, this probably varies with each patient according to their genetic risk and the environmental factors they encounter.

WHAT IS GOING ON IN THE SKIN?

The skin in eczema sufferers is heavily infiltrated with immune cells. This includes activated T cells (Chapter 5) that are even seen in the apparently unaffected skin of these patients. In an acute exacerbation these cells produce allergic (Type 2) cytokine signals, but in more longstanding lesions they then also produce type 1 cytokines (Chapter 5), which perpetuate the chronic inflammation. T cells can become more activated to induce these signals when they come into contact with allergens or bacterial products, such as 'super antigens' (below). Other cells present in eczema include antigen-presenting cells, mast cells and eosinophils (Chapters 3 and 5). Although many patients also have IgE antibodies to allergens, the role of these antibodies in driving the disease is controversial. Eczema and dermatitis can generally be considered to be the result of more chronic 'cell-driven' inflammation rather than 'antibody-driven' reactions, which are usually more acute and short-lived. IgE may initiate allergen-triggered exacerbations, but then the T cells take over.

THE APPEARANCE

When the disease is 'active' during an exacerbation, the skin shows clear signs of inflammation (redness) and is almost always very itchy. Depending on the severity of the flare-up, it may also be scaly, crusty, or weepy. There are often small lumps ('papules') or tiny blisters ('vesicles'). As the disease settles, the redness and inflammation subside and skin can return to a normal appearance. However, microscopic examination reveals that the skin is not really normal, even in completely normal-looking skin. Between exacerbations many patients experience residual 'dryness' and the tendency for itching can persist. After recurrent bouts the skin can often become thickened and very rough. There is a wide variation in the severity, which also fluctuates over time.

THE DISTRIBUTION

The location of any rash can also give vital clues in the diagnosis. Although eczema can affect any area of the skin, it is typically worse in the skin creases around joints, particularly the inner elbow, behind the knees, around the ankles and wrists. In infancy it can be more extensive, affecting the limbs more extensively and extending over the face, chest, abdomen and back.

How it changes with age

As a rough rule we can say that eczema improves in most children; although those with more severe disease are likely to show persistence in to adult life. Skin lesions are usually most extensive in the first years of life, and both the extent (total area affected) and the severity tend to improve with age. Mild cases often resolve completely. Children with more severe eczema are more likely to show persistent skin disease and to develop food allergies in the first years of life. They are also at greater risk of subsequent asthma and allergic rhinitis.

The symptoms

Itching is the main symptom. If there is no itch, it is unlikely that the rash is eczema.

The impact

The impact of chronic itching is far from trivial, at any age. Infants with eczema can be unsettled and irritable. Frequent waking at night is distressing and disruptive to the whole family. Extra time spent applying ointments and moisturisers every day places additional demands on family life. Older children and adults can also be very troubled and self-conscious about the appearance of the rash, especially on exposed areas such as the face, hands and limbs. Eczema can also have considerable economic impact, for both individuals and health care systems.

The diagnosis

There is no laboratory test for eczema. The diagnosis is based on the symptoms, appearance and the distribution of the rash. To qualify as eczema the rash must be itchy with a typical appearance and other suggestive features such as dryness, skin crease involvement, early age of onset, and/or a history (or family history) of other allergic disease.[6]

THE TRIGGERS

It is useful to identify triggers, as avoiding these may be helpful in controlling the disease and preventing flares. There are a number of well-recognised triggers. Certain clothing can irritate the skin. Woollen fibres can be abrasive. This is also seen when infants crawl on carpets. Nylon and synthetic materials do not 'breathe' as well as natural fibres and can flare eczema by allowing the skin to get over heated. Detergents and soaps can dehydrate the skin and remove the protective lipids (oils). This can cause irritation and directly disrupt the skin barrier integrity. Other chemicals and irritants can have the same effect. Allergens can be important triggers, but only for a subgroup of patients who react to a specific allergen. Avoidance of specific allergens is not justified unless there is a history of exacerbation with the allergen. Other factors, such as physical or emotional stress, have been associated with exacerbations, probably because of their potential effects on immune function.

THE ROLE OF SKIN BACTERIA

Bacteria are normally found on our skin, especially those from the *Staphylococcus* ('Staph') family. These are on everyone's skin and don't usually cause a problem unless the skin gets broken, numbers get too high, or more hostile strains move in.

People with eczema have much higher levels of the potentially more aggressive staph species *(Staphylococcus aureus)*. These bacteria can more easily bind and establish themselves in eczema; partly because eczema skin is deficient in antimicrobial defense products and partly because the skin barrier is less effective. The bacteria then make the skin disease worse by producing toxins that activate the T cells and drive more inflammation. These toxins are sometimes called 'super antigens' because of their capacity to activate almost *all* T cells they come in contact with (unlike normal antigens which only activate the small number of T cells which recognise them). Worse still, these toxins can interfere with the effectiveness of eczema treatments (such as steroid creams). Interestingly, people with eczema also make IgE antibodies against these staph super antigens. There is no clear evidence that these antibodies help reduce Staph levels, and this response may actually make the inflammation worse. So, even without causing signs of infection, the Staph aureus species can be a major contributor to the severity of eczema. This is why patients with eczema can respond very well to antimicrobial treatments.

SUSCEPTIBILITY TO MORE SERIOUS INFECTIONS

The defective skin barrier and defense mechanisms also mean that people with eczema are more vulnerable to other infections including fungi and viruses. Although uncommon, eczema can increase the risk of herpes infections (such as the common cold sore) becoming more extensive and widespread. This can be very serious and urgent and aggressive medical treatment is important when this typically localised infection starts to show signs of rapid spread. This looks quite different to normal eczema. The lesions may be painful, blistered and oozing, and the patient usually becomes very unwell. If this is suspected, it is important to seek urgent medical attention as this can become life threatening.

GENERAL PRINCIPLES OF TREATMENT

A good understanding of the disease is probably the most important aspect of managing it. It is important that patients/parents understand the chronic nature of eczema so they have realistic expectations of what they can achieve.

The main objectives of managing eczema are 1) to have a have a daily regime for keeping the disease under control and reduce exacerbations and 2) have a clear treatment plan for getting exacerbations under control when they do occur.

Daily control

Avoiding triggers is a major part of keeping the tendency for inflammation under control. This means avoiding detergents, soaps, perfumes and other irritants. Scratching or rubbing against abrasive surfaces can also exacerbate eczema. Certain clothing (wool fibres) can be abrasive and others (some synthetic materials) can make the skin sweaty and hot. Any extreme temperature changes can be irritating. As allergens can exacerbate eczema in some patients, it is useful to identify these as part of a targeted avoidance plan (below). There are also several simple strategies that can reduce the levels of skin bacteria, including the use of bleach baths several times per week (below).

Daily use of moisturisers is the other mainstay of preventive treatment. This means adding oils to baths and using aqueous creams as soap substitutes.[7] This soothes the skin, reduces dryness and helps restore the natural skin barrier. It can also reduce the desire to scratch. There are many products to choose from, and if a new product causes increased itching or burning sensations it should be discontinued. One of the more suitable moisturisers is soft white paraffin.[8] This is best applied immediately after a bath when the skin is still wet and warm.

Treating an acute exacerbation

Exacerbations are inevitable. The most effective way of getting these under control is using anti-inflammatory ointments on the affected areas, where there are signs of redness and inflammation. To be effective they need to be used regularly as prescribed until the inflammation subsides. Ointments are generally more effective than creams because they are thicker, more moisturising and stick to the skin better.

Most of these anti-inflammatory products are steroids. A major part of eczema education is reassurance that these products are safe when used as medically directed. As these are only being applied 'topically' (directly to the skin) they have an excellent safety profile compared to the side effects of oral (ingested) steroids. Many parents are also worried that topical steroids can cause skin damage and thinning of the skin. However, there is little cause for these fears if steroids are used appropriately for short periods.[9] Ironically, the problem is rather that 'steroid phobia' can lead to under-treatment, poor control and increased risk of persistent skin damage.

There are varying steroid potencies available allowing the treatment to be individualised according to symptoms. Patients with mild disease respond very quickly to weaker steroids, without the need for stronger preparations. Stronger steroids are reserved for more severe disease.

The aim is to get the inflammation under control as soon as possible. In patients prone to significant symptoms, it is preferable to apply moderate or strong steroids at the first signs of inflammation because these patients respond more quickly to those than to weak steroids. The dose can then be tapered down (rather than stopped abruptly), to reduce a rebound exacerbation of symptoms. With this approach the total dose of steroid can actually be much less than if a milder steroid is applied over a longer period of time.

There are newer alternatives to steroids that inhibit inflammation by suppressing T cell function ('calcineurin inhibitors'). These drugs (tacrolimus and pimecrolimus) are also applied as ointments and creams, and do not have the same side-effects as steroids. They are used in acute eczema treatment and to prevent flaring in more severe cases of the disease particularly in areas of the body that can be more sensitive to the effects of steroids such as the face, around the eyes and in the groin. Because they are less well studied, there are still some uncertainties about their effectiveness compared to steroids as well as their long-term safety.

A simple and effective way of getting on top of an acute exacerbation can be to apply these treatments (most typically steroids) under 'wet wraps' (described in more detail below).

Other treatments that can be useful during an acute exacerbation include antihistamines (for itch) and antibiotics (in severe exacerbations particularly if there is evidence of infection).

CASE STUDY

James was first referred to our clinic when he was fourteen months old. He had had eczema since he was two months old with frequent flares affecting large areas of his body. His family doctor had previously prescribed a mild 1% hydrocortisone cream for his face and a stronger one for his body. James's mother, Jenny, had been worried about using these and had not applied them consistently. She did use a moisturiser every day but could not get the flare-ups properly under control. He scratched constantly and woke crying almost every night. His sheets were often streaked with blood from his repeated scratching. Jenny was also very stressed and had tried excluding a range of foods from his diet including cow's milk, eggs and wheat. He once had a blotchy rash shortly after eating egg, but no other symptoms. This diet only had limited effect. When we first saw him, James had widespread, inflamed eczema with infected areas. He was very agitated and Jenny felt she could not cope much longer. Allergy testing (SPT) showed IgE sensitisation to egg (7 mm) and house dust mites (5 mm) but was negative to milk, wheat and other foods.

He was admitted to the ward for twice daily 'wet-wraps' and intensive topical steroid treatment using ointments rather than creams. Tacrolimus ointment was used on his face. This was followed by generous coverage of soft white paraffin moisturiser after his wraps. He was prescribed a course of oral antibiotics to treat the infected areas. He showed a dramatic improvement and within three days, Jenny said 'his skin never look so good'. She was given eczema education and her fears about using steroid products were addressed. She was taught how to use wet wraps at home and continued these daily for the remainder of the week and every second day for another seven days. We gave information on controlling house dust mite levels and advised her to continue excluding eggs from his diet. After things had settled down for a few weeks, Jenny was asked to try reintroducing cow's milk. The day after the milk James had another flare, and she was then advised to avoid all dairy products, with the help of our dietician. Jenny became more confident treating his flares and got them under control more quickly. A month later she reintroduced wheat, which he tolerated without an eczema flare. In the six months that followed James continued to have low-grade itchy patches and periodic flares. He was also still prone to skin infections. We advised Jenny to try diluted bleach bathes several times a week. He significantly improved after this with a general improvement in his skin and fewer flares. By the time he was three, he was tolerating egg in well-cooked foods and his egg SPT was only weakly positive (3 mm). He had developed occasional wheezing with colds and was suspected to be developing asthma. His eczema continues to improve with age.

POINTS THIS CASE ILLUSTRATES

- The stress and family disruption can be considerable
- Unwarranted fear of using medications, especially steroids, can lead to poor control and unnecessary symptoms
- Ointments are thicker, more moisturising and generally better than creams
- Wet wraps can improve the effectiveness of treatment and can be done at home
- Non-steroid anti-inflammatory ointments (such as tacrolimus) can be used on sensitive areas such as the face
- James also has IgE egg allergy, which is common in infants with eczema. His IgE symptoms are only mild but this could be a possible eczema trigger
- Although James does not have IgE milk allergy (SPT negative) he does have delayed symptoms suggesting a non-IgE reaction that appears to trigger his eczema

- Bleach added to the bath (in safe concentrations – see below) can improve eczema by reducing the levels of 'Staph' bacteria
- Children with eczema are prone to asthma and other allergies
- House dust mite, particularly in his bedding, could be a potential trigger for James's eczema because he is sensitised to mites.

WET WRAPS: A SIMPLE AND PRACTICAL STRATEGY

This is a very useful way to help steroid ointments penetrate and work more efficiently when eczema is flaring, widespread or severe. Wet wraps can feel very soothing to itchy skin. The idea is to bath and apply steroid ointment, then to apply a layer of warm wet clothing with a dry layer on top. In infants this can be a wet jump suit before wrapping them in a dry towel. It is important to keep the child warm in cool weather. Older children and adults with widespread eczema can use wet pyjamas with a dry dressing gown or track suit on top. After 20–30 minutes the wet garments are removed and moisturiser applied. For localised areas (such as the hands, feet or ankles) the same approach is used with wet cotton socks over the affected areas and dry socks over the top. Socks with the ends cut off can also be used over the knees and elbows. This is best done daily, at night when it can be relaxing and soothing before sleep. Once the skin has cleared, we often recommend continuing every second night for a week to consolidate the improvement.

BLEACH BATHS: ANOTHER SIMPLE AND EFFECTIVE STRATEGY

Many people are quite surprised when we suggest using bleach. Bleach (sodium hypochlorite) is used in cleaning products and dental antiseptic because it kills bacteria. The reason that this can be so effective in eczema is that it reduces *Staphylococcus aureus* bacteria on the skin, which can be a driving force in eczema exacerbations. A US study found that children with eczema who had dilute bleach baths combined with an antimicrobial ointment to the nose, had a marked improvement in the severity of eczema over the following months.[10]

Clearly bleach must be used at a dilute and safe concentration, so it is important to get the recipe right. In our clinic we use standard house hold bleach, which is generally around 4% sodium hypochlorite (40–42g/L). It is vital to check the concentration before using. We add 50 ml of this to a bathtub containing 40 litres of water (4 x 10 litres buckets), and recommend bathing for five–ten minutes twice weekly. Any more than that can be irritating to the skin. If there is extensive involvement of the upper body, we suggest wearing an old t-shirt in the bath and wetting it in the bath water.

It is also common to silently carry 'Staph' in the nose. This does not cause symptoms, but acts as a reservoir for recolonising the skin after eradication. The best 'anti-Staph' regimes therefore also use antibacterial ointment (containing mupirocin) in the nostrils twice a day for five consecutive days each month.

THE ROLE OF ALLERGENS IN ECZEMA

Many patients are sensitised to allergens, especially those with more severe symptoms. In early childhood when food allergy is most common (Chapter 11) food allergy can trigger eczema flares. This is suspected if there is a relationship between the food exposure and symptoms. While avoiding triggering foods can bring about improvement, it may not lead to complete resolution because eczema is usually multifactorial.

In IgE-mediated food allergy, the immediate symptoms of food allergy are usually obvious but can then give way to the more chronic symptoms of eczema. This is usually confirmed by IgE allergy tests to specific foods (Chapters 10 and 11). Avoidance is recommended for foods that are associated with any symptoms including eczema flares (Chapter 11). Positive allergy tests (i.e. SPT or RAST) do not necessarily indicate that food will cause food allergy or eczema flares. If there is no history of immediate reactions, these patients may require a trial elimination of food followed by a rechallenge to confirm if there is a relationship between the food and the eczema.

There are also children who show non-IgE mediated skin reactions to food. These children can show a flare in eczema more than twenty-four hours after eating the food. Allergy tests are negative and the reaction is believed to be T cell mediated. These children do not show signs of more serious IgE-mediated symptoms (Chapter 11), and because the reaction is delayed, the relationship can be harder to identify. When this is suspected a trial elimination of the food (for at least two–four weeks) is recommended, anticipating an improvement within two weeks if the food is a major trigger.[11] This should be followed by a food challenge to confirm that re-exposure induces exacerbation. If there is no change in the eczema during this process, it is hard to justify continued avoidance.

Foods are much less likely eczema triggers in older children and rare in adult-onset eczema. However, other allergens, such as house dust mite, can play a role. One of the preferred habitats for dust mites is our bedding, where they come in direct contact with the skin. This is a likely route of sensitisation in eczema patients, and once sensitised, dust mites can be a trigger for symptoms. These patients have positive IgE tests to the mites. Strategies to reduce mite levels can be worth a try, but this is often difficult (Chapter 13). In patients where dust mites are suspected to be a major trigger, and the symptoms are bad enough, immunotherapy can be considered (Chapter 10).

THE END OF THE LINE: WHEN NOTHING ELSE WORKS

Some patients have very severe and resistant disease, which does not respond to all these measures. Fortunately, this is only a small proportion of all people with eczema. These patients may need much more aggressive treatment with oral immune suppressive drugs, ultraviolet B (light) therapy, or even gamma globulin (IgG antibody) infusions. These treatments should only be used in very severe disease and must be done under the guidance of experienced specialists.

THE PROGNOSIS

The outlook for eczema very much depends on the severity. Most young children have mild disease that will resolve during childhood. However, those with more severe disease are more likely to show persistence into adulthood. For these families it is about coping rather than finding a cure, at least for now. We can control the disease but as yet we cannot yet reverse the underlying causes. But every year, a better understanding of the condition brings us steadily closer.

• • •

Our skin provides an essential physical barrier to protect us from the environment. There are also resident immune cells, specialised antigen presenting cells (APC, Chapter 5) which patrol for invaders, poised to call in the T cells at the first signs of trouble. In normal skin, most of the time things are quiet. The roaming sentinel APC don't have much to report, and T cells stay deployed elsewhere. But in eczema things are very different. The physical barrier is less effective. Foreign proteins and irritants can penetrate more easily. The APC work overtime calling armies of T cells to take occupation. When they do, they are more likely to initiate Type 2 allergic responses to perceived threats whether these are harmful or not.

New understanding of the driving influences behind these events may provide new strategies for treatment. Recent identification of genetic mutations in skin barrier components has shed new light on the importance of the physical barrier, possibly even as the initiating event in some patients. In other patients the immune propensity for allergy may be the driving factor that then contributes to a breakdown of the skin barrier. Which ever happens first, both processes are contributory and it is likely that new treatments will target both the skin barrier and the immune response.

13

Asthma

Fighting for each breath. Suffocating from the inside. Fear. Exhaustion. No control. That is how people with asthma can feel as their airways tighten and narrow down. This can be a frightening condition, which still has no cure. The impact of asthma took a more palpable and personal meaning for me in medical school when a close friend lost his mother to asthma. He helplessly watched her die at home before help could arrive. Gasping for air. But her airways were so tight she could not even inhale her medications. It was horrific. That was in the 1980s and treatment to control asthma has improved since then, but asthma remains a serious and potentially life threatening condition.

Just like all of the other conditions associated with the allergy epidemic, asthma has shown a dramatic rise in incidence. The World Health Organisation has estimated that around 300 million people worldwide have asthma, and that 250,000 die prematurely each year from asthma.[1] With almost all of these deaths avoidable, the World Allergy Organization (WAO) is playing a major role in promoting awareness, funding, education and research into better asthma and allergy care.[2]

Currently, in high prevalence industrialised countries more than 20 per cent of school age children have had symptoms of asthma.[3] It is one of the best-studied conditions among the disorders associated with allergy. This is because asthma has an enormous impact on health and society and because it was one of the early signs of the allergy epidemic, predating the more recent rise in food allergy. Although there is some evidence that asthma rates may have reached a plateau in some countries,[4] rates are continuing to rise in less developed regions[5] as these regions adopt an urbanised western lifestyle. Although there is no cure, there has been significant progress in improving symptoms control and quality of life for patients with asthma.

WHAT IS IT?

Asthma is caused by inflammation of the small airways. This inflammation leads to swelling, mucous secretion and involuntary contraction of the muscle fibres within these small airways. Together, these changes all contribute to the narrowing and obstruction of the airway that culminate in an asthma 'attack' or acute exacerbation. Over the longer term, repeated inflammation and airway damage can lead to abnormal healing. Instead of repairing to their normal state, scar tissue forms and the airway muscles get bigger so that narrowing with future exacerbations can be even greater. This abnormal repair is often called 'airway remodelling'.

As with the skin in eczema, asthma is also the result of both local events in the airways and systemic (generalised) immune events, which predispose to airways inflammation. This is another complex condition that is the culmination of a number of genetic and environmental factors. These can vary widely between individuals. In a waiting room full of asthmatics, we could expect to find many different genetic profiles and different patterns of environmental exposures. Not surprisingly, we also see a wide range in the severity, frequency and patterns of symptoms over time. This is why asthma is *not* a 'single' condition, but rather airways inflammation that may have a number of different origins. Accordingly, we also need to individualise treatment.

The role of genetics in asthma

The most obvious evidence of a genetic role is that asthma runs in families. Having an immediate family member with asthma is a recognised risk factor. There are a large number of genes that have been linked with asthma, but no single gene that is common to all asthmatics (Chapter 7). This suggests that a range of genes can contribute to asthma and that these can vary between individuals. Genes that have been linked with asthma include genetic variants (polymorphisms, Chapter 7) in airway remodelling genes, IgE receptor genes, Type 2 cytokine genes, and other immune genes. Having any or all of these gene variants increases the risk of asthma, but does not mean the disease will definitely develop.

Environmental factors that may contribute to the development of asthma

The environmental factors that can trigger attacks of asthma (such as viral infections, allergens, smoking and other pollutants), may also play a role in initiating the disease in the first place (Chapter 8).

One of the best-known risk factors for infant wheezing and asthma is cigarette smoking. Maternal smoking in pregnancy can alter airways development and immune function (Chapter 8). Other exposures in pregnancy may also influence early immune development to increase the risk of allergic airways inflammation after birth. After birth, viral chest infections are a risk factor for asthma, although this relationship is complex (Chapter 8).

The role of allergy in asthma

Allergic immune responses are a strong risk factor for the development of asthma. Once asthma is established, allergens can also trigger exacerbations in sensitised patients. Many asthmatics show Type 2 immune responses and IgE production against allergens. The airways of asthmatics also show infiltration with Type 2 T cells, eosinophils and mast cells which all drive allergic inflammation (Chapters 3 and 5). Allergic sensitisation to inhaled allergens (such as house dust mite) is also a risk for the progression or persistence of asthma. In patients who do have allergy, treating the allergy (with immunotherapy) can improve the asthma; a clear indication that allergy and asthma are interrelated. However, not all asthmatics are allergic. As for eczema (Chapter 12) this indicates that allergy is a risk factor, but not essential for asthma to develop.

TRIGGERS

Common triggers of acute asthma attacks include viral infection, allergen exposure, cold air, exercise, cigarette smoke and other irritants. In some patients gastro-oesophageal (acid) reflux disease can also be a trigger. Asthma is a 'pattern of response' when these triggers are encountered. Once that response pattern has been established in the airways and in the immune system, the final effect will be roughly the same regardless of the trigger.

SIGNS AND SYMPTOMS OF AN ACUTE ATTACK

The symptoms of asthma all reflect the narrowing and obstruction of airways by muscle tightening and secretions. This includes tightness of the chest, coughing, secretions (sputum) and wheezing, which is the noise of airflow through constricted air tubes.

The signs (what we see when we look at someone with acute asthma) also reflect the obstruction. To understand this best, is it useful to consider the exact location of the obstruction. We can think of the airways like the branches of a tree, with the main air pipe (trachea) leading to smaller branches (bronchi and the twig-like bronchioles) and eventually out to the tiny air sacs (alveoli) where the oxygen exchange occurs. Asthma mainly affects the small branches of these airways. During an attack, the increased effort to draw air into the chest can be seen as the softer tissues (between the ribs and at the base of the throat) get sucked in.

This may not be noticeable in very mild attacks. In more severe exacerbations, this retraction can be quite visible and is best seen in oblique light when shadows make it more obvious. The rate of breathing also increases. So does the heart rate. When patients are working very hard to breathe they may lift their shoulders in an extra effort to get more air. These can be signs that the attack is very severe. Ironically, if anything, the chest actually looks *full* of air (hyper-inflated). This is because the narrowing of the smaller air tubes causes 'air trapping' beyond in the air sacs. After getting the air in it is even harder to squeeze it out again. This is also why the 'wheezing' sound is heard more during exhaling. We can contrast this to what happens with anaphylaxis (Chapter 11) where obstruction in the upper airways (outside the chest) causes noisy breathing ('stridor') more when inhaling.

Despite the increased effort, this can still be insufficient to achieve enough airflow which leads to a drop in the oxygen levels reaching the blood. A subtle reduction in oxygen levels is not visible, but as the levels drop further the lips can appear 'dusky' with a blue hue ('cyanosis'). The heart rate increases further. In very severe cases, patients become exhausted, unable to maintain the increased work of breathing. When obstruction is critical, the wheezing may actually be less audible because airflow is so limited. In this situation a 'silent' chest is a very worrying sign. Without treatment, very severe attacks can be fatal. But these days it rarely comes to that. Better control of the inflammation reduces the risk of attacks and early treatment of an attack can bring it under control before it gets this severe.

SIGNS AND SYMPTOMS OF ASTHMA *BETWEEN* ATTACKS

When we are assessing asthma severity and asthma 'control', we are just as interested (sometimes more so) in how the patient is *between* episodes. This gives vital clues to whether there is continuing inflammation that needs ongoing treatment.

Many patients with mild asthma have no symptoms at all between episodes. Others have persistent or intermittent low-grade symptoms that reflect ongoing inflammation of the airways. This can be as subtle as only coughing at night or after exercise, and this may not be recognised as asthma at all. Or there may be other more obvious symptoms, such as wheezing and a feeling of chest tightness. These niggling symptoms don't necessarily lead to a full-blown exacerbation, but are a sign that the inflammation is not adequately controlled and regular medications may be needed. It is even possible to have these 'interval' symptoms without *ever* having had a full-blown asthma attack. In such patients the diagnosis may be missed or delayed.

Like the acute exacerbations, these 'interval' symptoms are the result of low-grade inflammation causing mucous secretion and muscle tightening in the airways. These airway muscles are not under our conscious control. We can't just relax them at will. They are very different from the muscles under our voluntary control. In asthmatics, these involuntary 'smooth' muscles are prone to becoming both over-developed and over-responsive or twitchy. Fortunately they usually respond well to medications that are effectively smooth muscle relaxants (or 'broncho-dilators') such as salbutamol.

There can be variations in symptoms over the course of the day, with some patients reporting worsening of symptoms at night and in the early morning. This reflects normal body rhythms. Our bodies make natural steroid hormones (in our adrenal glands). These are essential for life and have anti-inflammatory properties among their many other functions. Levels normally drop to a low point in the early hours of the morning. This is why symptoms of inflammation of the airways can be worse at this time, when the body's 'internal' anti-inflammatory system is at low ebb.

ALL THAT WHEEZES IS NOT ASTHMA

A wheeze is caused by narrowing of the small airways. But this is not always caused by asthma. In young infants viral chest infections are the most common cause of wheezing. The virus causes swelling and secretions but generally without the smooth muscle tightening of asthma – so the bronchodilator muscle relaxant drugs do not usually help. At this young age, the airways are small and prone to narrowing to a level that causes difficulty breathing and results in the wheezing sound. This infection is called bronchiolitis which literally means inflammation of the small airways (bronchioles). It is self-resolving and most infants who wheeze with this viral infection do not have asthma and never will. But for a subgroup this can herald the beginning of viral-triggered asthma. The problem is discerning these. They can appear indistinguishable, and this is the reason that there is reluctance to label children with asthma too early. But there are clues. The likelihood that they are on the 'asthma-track' is greater if they have signs of other allergic disease (such as food allergy or eczema) or if there is a family history of asthma or any of these other conditions. Because it is difficult to make a diagnosis in these children, they should be observed with a suspicious eye. In time, the true asthmatics declare themselves. The more episodes there are like this, the more grounds for suspicion. A trial of bronchodilator asthma medication can be considered, and a response can clinch the diagnosis because this confirms smooth muscle tightening was contributing to the symptoms – in other words, asthma. Other causes of wheeze in infants include cystic fibrosis, structural abnormalities, and inhaled small objects (which get lodged in an airway) or milk during feeding. These conditions usually have other features that help distinguish them from asthma.

DIAGNOSING ASTHMA

There is no exact way to diagnose asthma, meaning that we might arrive at the same diagnosis differently depending on the patient.

In each case, this is usually based on varying combinations of history, symptoms, physical signs (if there are any at the time of consultation) and investigations. In many cases, the history alone can be highly suggestive of asthma. We usually like to confirm wheezing and other physical signs by examining the patient's chest during an episode, but the absence of physical signs (or an opportunity to check for these) does not exclude a diagnosis of asthma. Lung function tests can also be highly useful for demonstrating airflow limitation and responsiveness to bronchodilators. These tests generally require active blowing into a machine, which measures a range of breathing parameters including the rate of airflow and the lung capacity. Different lung diseases show characteristic patterns. In asthma, the main abnormality is restricted airflow during exhalation due to the narrowing of the smaller air tubes. This test involves the patient taking a deep breath and then exhaling as hard and fast as possible into a machine that measures the airflow, and this can be difficult for children under six or seven years of age. When asthma is suspected in younger children, (based on the history of recurrent or persistent wheeze) it is usually confirmed by an improvement in these symptoms after a trial of bronchodilator treatment. Chest X-rays are not routine, but may be useful if the diagnosis is not clear, of if the symptoms suggest other conditions or complications of asthma.

CLASSIFYING ASTHMA SEVERITY

Classifying the severity helps determine the best treatment approach. This classification needs to reflect the underlying control of asthma between attacks rather than just the severity of the attacks. It is also important that we regularly reassess asthma control as this can change over time, and can indicate that treatment requirements also need to change. A number of different classifications have been used but most of these take into account the frequency and persistence of symptoms, whether there are symptoms at night (sleep disturbance) and the level of lung function impairment (in older children and adults). The classification outlined here is based on a sentinel evidence-based document[6] prepared using extensive evaluation of all relevant international research, with due consideration of recommendations of other international expert bodies including 'GINA' the Global Initiative for Asthma <www.ginaasthma.com> and the British Thoracic Society <www.brit-thoracic.org.uk>. These are a dynamic, updated every few years as more evidence comes to light. They are highly practical documents, made available on-line for primary care givers around the world. I was fortunate to be involved as a member of the working-group involved in preparing the current version (2011) of the *Asthma Management Handbook*. We worked closely with other experts and our National Asthma Council <www.nationalasthma.org.au>, to ensure that issues relating to the 'allergic aspects' of this disease were included with more emphasis than in earlier documents.[7]

Intermittent asthma

Fortunately, the majority of asthmatics fall into this category. This includes patients with mild asthma who rarely have any symptoms between exacerbations, and when they do these are brief (usually mild) and infrequent (less than every four–six weeks). Children are sometimes further defined as 'frequent' intermittent asthma sufferers if their exacerbations happen more often. If the lung function can be measured (depending on age) in patients with intermittent asthma usually show fairly good or normal function (more than 80 per cent of predicted levels).

Persistent asthma

Patients who do have regular symptoms between exacerbations, more than once a week during the day or at night, have persistent asthma. These can be further classified as '*mild* persistent', '*moderate* persistent' or '*severe* persistent' depending on how much this is restricting physical activity, sleep and lung function.

GENERAL PRINCIPLES OF TREATMENT

The key aims are to treat acute attacks (exacerbations) quickly and effectively and then to improve asthma control between exacerbations, which will improve lung function and reduce the risk of future attacks.[8]

Treatment of acute asthma

All children and adults with known asthma should be prescribed short-acting bronchodilator 'reliever' inhalers (such as salbutamol) to treat an exacerbation as soon as the symptoms begin. Most countries now have standardised 'Asthma Action Plans' with specific instructions on how do so this. Although many people think that 'nebuliser' machines are the best way to give bronchodilators during an exacerbation, this is not true. The most efficient way of giving the asthma medication is actually using the 'puffer' inhaler with a 'spacer' device, which is a container with a hole at either in; one to attach the puffer and the other to breathe through (see 'Devices' page 196). This effectively suspends the particles so they can be inhaled. It also delivers the dose more quickly than a nebuliser. So, faced with an acute attack, giving six to twelve puffs of a bronchodilator through the spacer is as effective as a nebuliser. Most emergency centres now only reserve nebulisers for very severe attacks requiring continuous medication.

In most mild to moderate exacerbations, the bronchodilator dose can be repeated at home every three to four hours as required until symptoms settle. If the symptoms do not improve or the medication is needed more often, the patient should be assessed in an emergency centre where the bronchodilator may be needed more frequently. The patient can be more closely monitored and oxygen given as necessary. A short course of oral steroids such as prednisolone is often prescribed (for several days) to get significant exacerbations under control quickly. In more severe cases, the steroid may be given intravenously along with other medications to control the symptoms. Fortunately, this is only required in a small minority of cases.

Treatment between exacerbations

There are many aspects to improving asthma control between exacerbations, including minimising triggering factors and providing additional medications if they are indicated. This needs to be tailored to each patient's individual situation and requirements. Some triggers should be universally avoided (such as cigarette smoke) whereas others (such as allergens) will vary with the sensitisation profile (see below). As viral infections are common asthma triggers influenza vaccinations are often recommended in asthma patients, especially those with persistent asthma. Good education for self-management (or for caregivers in children) is essential for optimal asthma control.

Patients with infrequent intermittent asthma do not need any asthma medications between episodes. They just need to make sure their bronchodilator is ready in case they develop an exacerbation.

On the other hand, patients with more persistent asthma are likely to need a daily 'preventer' medication.[9] In general this applies to any patient with symptoms more than three times a week.[10] That is the reason we often ask if patients need to use their 'reliever' bronchodilator treatment more than three times a week. Other indications for considering preventer medications include poor lung function, and frequent and severe exacerbations.

The choice of daily preventer depends on the severity of the asthma, especially in children. Generally, inhaled steroids are still the most effective medication for achieving and maintaining asthma control in adults and in children with persistent asthma. However, in children with only 'mild persistent' asthma or 'frequent inter-mittent' asthma, there can be a choice between low dose inhaled steroids, a non-steroid 'cromone' inhaler, or a chewable tablet (that blocks inflammatory leuktrienes, Chapter 3). But in more severe disease (moderate and severe persistent asthma) the inhaled steroids remain the preferred choice.

Ideally, patients should be reassessed two–three months after starting a new treatment to see if the control is adequate. Once the asthma is stable and controlled, it is ideal to step down the dose of inhaled steroids to the minimum effective dose. If the control is not adequate it may be necessary to increase the dose of steroid or to add in another 'symptom controller' medication. Symptom controllers are usually long-acting bronchodilators that can help reduce symptoms. Because their benefits last longer, they are particularly useful in reducing symptoms through the night. These symptom controllers are often combined with a steroid in a single device and referred to as a 'combination' treatment which is available in different dose combinations. Again, once asthma is controlled, it is recommended that treatment doses be stepped down. Adding a long-acting bronchodilator may also ultimately allow lower doses of inhaled steroid.

Other immune modifying treatments (such as immuno-therapy) can be beneficial but are usually reserved for patients with persistent asthma (see below) where allergens are a significant trigger.

Treating symptoms with exercise
Many patients have symptoms following exercise, ranging from mild coughing and wheezing to a full-blown attack. Symptoms often become worse five–ten minutes *after* they stop exercising. This is really just another indicator that asthma is not under con-trol optimal, and ideally should be confirmed on lung function tests. Adding an asthma preventer (such as inhaled steroids or

anti-leukotriene tablets) can improve control, especially if there are other symptoms of persistent asthma control. Patients also benefit from the use of a short-acting bronchodilator immediately before they start exercising. Long-acting bronchodilators are also used, but these are best used intermittently because their protection against exercise-induced asthma can be reduced when they are taken daily.

CASE STUDY

Joshua is a two and a half year old boy, referred for recurrent wheezing with colds. He first wheezed at six months of age and was diagnosed with mild bronchiolitis. He did not require any specific treatment and recovered completely. He had some mild eczema that has been improving with age and his older sister has asthma. About five months later he had another similar episode, again mild, and which did not require any treatment. At that stage he had no symptoms between episodes. On his third episode at eighteen months of age, his wheezing was more pronounced and his family doctor decided to try a 'reliever' bronchodilator treatment through a spacer with a mask. Joshua's wheezing clearly improved. The doctor prescribed a three-day course of oral steroids and Joshua's mother continued the bronchodilator treatment at home every four–six hours until his symptoms resolved four days later. She was advised to try the reliever whenever Joshua had episodes of wheezing and coughing. More recently she has noticed that Joshua is coughing more at night and occasionally wakes from sleep with wheezing. She has also heard him coughing more after he has been running around. She has found the reliever bronchodilator helps and has been using it four–five times each week. Based on this, his doctor started a trial of an inhaled steroid preventer twice daily, every day. Within two weeks his mother noticed that his night symptoms had completely settled. Since starting the preventer, Joshua has had several colds without developing any wheezing. As most of his symptoms occur in winter, he will continue the preventer throughout until early summer when there is a plan to reduce his dose or trial him off the preventer over summer. Although his older sister is allergic to house dust mites and grass pollens, so far Joshua's allergy tests have been negative.

Points this case illustrates

- Viral illnesses are the most common trigger for asthma in young children
- Many infants can wheeze with viral illnesses and not have asthma. This can make it difficult to diagnose asthma in the first years of life. Joshua has other risk factors (a family history of asthma and eczema, which make it more likely that his wheezing may indeed be asthma)
- Bronchodilators are not used in very young infants with viral wheezing, because they do not usually help and may make symptoms worse (especially in children under six months)
- In older infants who have had recurrent wheezing, trial of a bronchodilator treatment is helpful for diagnosing asthma if there is an improvement in symptoms
- A spacer with a mask is the best way of giving inhaled treatments at this age
- Initially Joshua appeared to have infrequent intermittent symptoms, and he did not require any treatment between episodes
- More recently he has developed more persistent symptoms which required preventer treatment. This highlights the need for regular review as disease patterns can change
- He responded well and there is a plan to reduce his dose of regular steroids as tolerated
- Allergens do not play a major role in Joshua's symptoms, but he is at risk of sensitisation as he gets older.

The delivery device is just as important as the drug

Medications will not work if they are not given properly. Having the right device at the right age and using it properly are all central to good asthma management. The best way of delivering asthma medications is directly where they are needed: inhaled into the airways. Surprisingly, it was not that long ago that bronchodilator treatment was given orally in syrup to young infants. Clearly this was less effective and produced more side-effects than when the same drugs are delivered directly to the lungs. Now we have better ways of delivering asthma drugs directly into the lungs, but many patients do not use the devices correctly.

The most common error is the use of asthma 'puffers' without a spacer device. Spacers should generally always be used for any pressurised metered dose inhaler (such as during the treatment of acute asthma symptoms), especially in children. Without the spacer, a high proportion of the medication hits the back of the throat and does not reach the chest; even in coordinated adults who can inhale at the same time as activating the puffer spray. This significantly reduces the effectiveness of the medication. Spacers have valves to ensure the air flows in one direction and they come in varying sizes. The smaller volume spacers used in younger children (two–four years) usually have a face mask attached. Larger volume spacers (without masks) are used in older children and adults. The respiratory unit at my hospital (the Children's Hospital in Perth) has also done research which showed this simple technique is more efficient than using nebulisers,[11] which are expensive, cumbersome and more difficult to maintain. Because most spacers are plastic, a static electricity charge can reduce delivery. This is overcome by simply washing the spacer in warm water and kitchen detergent then allowing the device to air-dry *without* rinsing. This is done before the first use and then at least once a month.[12]

There are newer devices that do not require spacers, which are more popular with teenagers and adults, named variously as autohalers, accuhalers or turbuhalers. These are 'breath-activated', and do not 'puff'. This means that delivery of the medication relies on the patient taking a deep breath to suck the medication down into the airways. Young children (generally under the age of seven or eight) cannot use these devices. A number of different asthma medications can be delivered through these breath-activated devices (including bronchodilators, preventers, symptom controllers and combination medications).

An important part of asthma management is education and training to make sure each patient can effectively use the device they are prescribed.

CASE STUDY

Sarah is Joshua's older sister. She is now twelve years old and, like her brother, has also has asthma since infancy. She has been on preventer steroid inhalers for a number of years, and has required a combination treatment more recently (inhaled steroid combined with a long-acting bronchodilator symptom-controller) to control her symptoms. Her allergy tests show that she is allergic to house dust mite and grass pollens. Sarah's asthma is often worse when she visits her grandmother's house, which is quite dusty. She also has allergic rhinitis and was started on a nasal steroid spray with the aim of improving both her nasal and her chest symptoms. Her mother has tried house dust mite reduction strategies (by covering Sarah's bedding with mite proof covers) with only partial improvement in her asthma and rhinitis. At school Sarah was using her 'puffer' without a spacer because she was embarrassed to use the spacer in front of her friends. She was using it before sport, but still had frequent exercise-induced symptoms. She has had two asthma exacerbations in the preceding six months, one requiring admission to hospital. Her lung function was about 75 per cent of her predicted level and this showed significant improvement following bronchodilator treatment. We changed her bronchodilator inhaler to a breath-activated device that can be used without a spacer. After much deliberation, Sarah and her family agreed to immunotherapy. She has had incremental increasing doses of house mite and grass extracts over several months and has been on her regular monthly maintenance injection for eight months now. Her rhinitis symptoms have improved significantly and her asthma control is much better. We have been able to reduce the dose of her steroid inhalers. Her exercise tolerance is improving although she still needs to use her bronchodilator occasionally. She was initially troubled by some local swelling over the injection site after her immunotherapy injection site, but this is now controlled by a non-sedating antihistamine a few hours before her dose. The plan is to continue her injections for a total of three years.

Points this case illustrates

- Sarah has moderate persistent asthma, with frequent symptoms and moderately severe exacerbations. Her disease is only partially controlled despite preventers and symptom controllers
- Using a puffer (metered dose inhaler) without a spacer may have contributed to its ineffectiveness in reducing Sarah's exercise symptoms
- Older children (and adults) can use newer 'breath-activated' devices that don't require spacers, and usually prefer to carry these as symptom relievers
- Asthma is often associated with allergic rhinitis. Inflammation in the upper airways (nose) can increase inflammation in the lower airways (asthma). Treatment of nasal inflammation has been shown to improve asthma control in some patients
- Allergens can be a significant trigger in older patients who are sensitised to that allergen
- Allergen reduction strategies can help in some patients, but they can be expensive, hard to implement and may not help in many patients
- It is important to minimise the total daily dose of steroid inhalers, especially in children. When a nasal steroid is also used (for allergic rhinitis) this should be included when calculating the total daily dose
- Adding other mediations (such as long-acting bronchodilator symptom controllers) may help reduce the steroid requirement while still maintaining asthma control
- Immunotherapy is a viable treatment option in persistent asthma, when symptoms are triggered by allergens and sensitisation to that allergen is confirmed
- There is good evidence that immunotherapy can improve asthma control and reduce steroid and other medication requirements
- In this case the immunotherapy was given by injection but it can also be given sublingually (under the tongue). The choice is based on cost, availability, likelihood of compliance and patient preference
- Injection immunotherapy should always be given under medical observation with resuscitation equipment available because of the risk

of reactions. Antihistamines before injection can reduce local side effects and do not interfere with the treatment effect.

SAFETY OF INHALED STEROIDS

It is always important to find the right balance between the benefits and risks of any medication for each patient. One of the main questions we are asked is 'are the inhaled steroids safe?' This is because, given orally for long periods of time, steroids have clear and recognised side effects. But they are virtually never given that way in asthma. Oral steroids are usually only given for very short periods (several days) to suppress an acute asthma attack. This is too short for any long-term effects to develop. When steroids are used for long-term control, they are given by the inhaled route at much lower doses. Given this way – delivered directly to the airways – even over long periods, the serious systemic effects of steroids are rarely seen. Local side effects, such as oral thrush, can be minimised by rinsing the mouth after inhaling each dose. However, it is always important that patients are on the lowest dose necessary to control their disease and that patients who do need higher doses are monitored closely for side effects, including osteoporosis, adrenal gland function and cataracts in adults.

Minimising the dose is particularly important in children who can be more sensitive to the effects. Although side effects are also uncommon in children at standard low doses of steroid preventers, higher doses can be associated with growth suppression. On the flip side, poorly controlled asthma can also cause growth suppression, in addition to long-term lung damage. This is one of the many reasons that height and lung function are monitored on a regular basis in most children's clinics. As ever, it is a question of balance. Fortunately for most children, their asthma is not severe enough to warrant higher doses of inhaled steroids. But when calculating the daily dose, it is important to include other steroids (such as nasal steroids in allergic rhinitis) in the total daily tally. In most cases adding other (non-steroid) preventers and symptom controllers can reduce the steroid requirement.

THE ROLE OF ALLERGY TESTING, ALLERGEN AVOIDANCE AND IMMUNOTHERAPY

Allergy testing is not necessary in every patient with asthma. It is most useful in patients where symptoms appear to be triggered by allergens, especially in patients with persistent asthma and in patients who also have other symptoms such as allergic rhinitis. Identifying allergen triggers can be helpful for targeted avoidance (if this is possible) or when immunotherapy is being considered as a treatment option.

Inhalant allergens are a major trigger for asthma in sensitised individuals. While this is less relevant in very young children who have not yet developed sensitisation, it often becomes an issue with age (as by school age around 40 per cent of all children in developed countries have evidence of inhalant sensitisations). The most common inhaled allergens include house dust mite, pollen, pets, moulds and cockroaches. These can trigger asthma attacks or make persistent symptoms worse – but *only* in sensitised individuals; and not all those sensitised will have symptoms on exposure. This is why the symptom history is so important.

In an ideal world, complete avoidance of allergens would prevent exacerbations, *if* this was possible and *if* allergens were the only trigger. But in the real world there are many other triggers and it is impossible to completely avoid allergens. Even reducing exposure to these allergens can be difficult. Because of this, there is no conclusive evidence that measures to reduce allergens (such as dust mite) will control asthma; however, some patients clearly do benefit from these strategies. The most simple of these strategies is to cover the bedding (pillows, quilts and mattresses) with dust mite proof covers. Detailed information is available on most allergy society websites. Although we provide this information, we also make families aware that these covers can be expensive and that they are not always effective.

Immunotherapy is a much more effective strategy for patients who have significant allergen-triggered asthma. There is good evidence that immunotherapy (Chapter 10) can modify allergic immune responses and lessen asthma, but this should only be used when allergens trigger symptoms and the patient's IgE allergy tests are proven to be positive for that allergen. Immunotherapy may be useful when there has been poor response to preventer medications, desire to reduce steroid requirements, and/or co-existing allergic rhinitis (Chapter 14). Because of the risk of reactions to immuno-therapy, it is generally not recommended in the small proportion of patients who have very severe and unstable asthma. As discussed in Chapter 10, immunotherapy is a significant undertaking, and patients need to be comfortable with and committed to the process. As always, the decision to undertake immunotherapy needs to be individualised based on the severity of symptoms, the likely benefits, the risks and the inconvenience of the treatment.

Although there are other immune therapies, these are very expensive and not widely available. These include antibody infusions to block the IgE cascade. They prevent the release of inflammatory mediators (histamines, leukotrienes, cytokines and others) by blocking the interaction of allergens with IgE on the surface of mast cells and other immune cells (Chapter 3). Unlike immunotherapy, these anti-IgE infusions do not permanently alter the immune response, but because they reduce the risk of IgE anaphylaxis, they may be used more in the future in conjunction with immunotherapy (and specific oral tolerance induction) to reduce reactions.

CONCEPT OF 'ONE AIRWAY': LINKS TO ALLERGIC RHINITIS

The nose and the lower airways are at either end of the same respiratory 'tree', so it is not surprising that asthma and rhinitis are strongly related (also discussed in Chapter 14). Similar immune processes drive these conditions and they often co-exist. People with allergic rhinitis have an increased future risk of developing asthma, if they don't have it already. Active inflammation in the nose can exacerbate asthma symptoms and treatment of the rhinitis can improve asthma symptoms. Many patients with asthma have sinus inflammation without realising it. For this reason we look for evidence of rhinitis in asthma patients, and make sure it is well treated (Chapter 14).

LINKS WITH FOOD ALLERGY

As food allergy and asthma are both a manifestation of the same allergic tendency, they are often related. Children with food allergy are much more likely to suffer from asthma. But food allergens are not common asthma triggers. Breathing difficulties associated with a food allergy reaction are more commonly due to anaphylaxis and should be treated with adrenaline (Chapter 12). Bronchodilator asthma drugs do not help anaphylaxis, even in asthmatics with food allergy. Using asthma treatments during anaphylaxis can delay the use of life-saving adrenaline, which should be the first treatment given when there are breathing difficulties after food ingestion. Most importantly, if patients with asthma *also* have anaphylactic food allergy, it is very important that the asthma is kept under good control; fatal anaphylaxis is more likely when asthma is poorly controlled.

★   ★   ★

We have moved ahead in leaps and bounds in improving the management of asthma, but not without enormous and continuing cost to our health systems globally. People do outgrow asthma, especially in early childhood, but this often happens whether we intervene or not, and many are not so lucky. Deaths from asthma might be much less common with better management and better control, but they still do occur. Our ultimate goal should still be to cure or, even better, to prevent this disease. In this, our progress has been much slower because there is so much we need to understand about this and other complex immune diseases. Fortunately asthma has been a priority area of research in many regions and this is helping us to gather the thousands of jigsaw pieces of this highly complex picture. The fact that the rise in asthma has been driven by the environmental change rather than genetics gives us cause for optimism that it may also be possible to reverse this one day.

14

Allergic rhinitis and allergic rhinoconjunctivitis

Can't breathe. Can't sleep. Can't concentrate. Head aches. Always tired. Itching. Sneezing. Snoring. Nose running. Dark rings under my eyes. Bad breath. Dry mouth. Embarrassed and self conscious. Bad behaviour and learning difficulties.

These are just some of the complaints of people with 'hayfever'. As a child, my teachers were always telling me to close my mouth and 'stop catching flies'. But they didn't seem to understand that I could not breathe any other way. At least not in the pollen season. Or around cats. Or dust. I was one of the first generations to experience the large-scale rise of hayfever. There was no doctor in our town. So the chemist gave me antihistamines, which sent me to sleep, and decongestants, which worked for a few hours. When they wore off I seemed to be even worse. Sometimes it was almost unbearable. Especially when my parents sent me to guitar lessons, where my teacher had a cat. They had already bought me a guitar, and when I refused to go, they decided to take my lessons instead. So my hayfever helped open the door on a new world for my parents. It was the 1970s, and not long before they became vegetarians and started wearing caftans. But that is another story.

Although allergic rhinitis is the most common allergic condition in many areas, it is often not taken seriously, regarded instead as trivial and inconvenient. But its effects are vastly underestimated.

It can significantly interfere with quality of life, productivity and performance at work or school. Because it is so common, it has a major impact on national health and economic costs in developed countries. For example, in Australia it is a major contributor to the estimated annual cost of allergic disease ($21.5 billion) in 2007, which was almost twice as large as those estimated for arthritis ($11.7 billion) or hearing loss ($11.7 billion), and far in excess of conditions such as schizophrenia ($1.8 billion) and bipolar disorder ($1.6 billion).[1] This report aptly indicated that the costs of allergic disease are not to be sneezed at!

WHAT IS IT?

The name 'hayfever' emerged in the nineteenth century when this condition was thought to be a contagious condition triggered by an unknown infectious agent carried in pollens and hay. That name still survives today even though we know it is neither contagious nor associated with fever. To our knowledge it was first described by British physician John Bostock in 1819 as a very rare and curious seasonal affliction that he suffered from.[2] In a national search over the ten years that followed, he found only twenty-eight similar cases.[3] All cases were in the middle and upper classes including 'some indeed of high rank'. He was at a complete loss to explain or treat this condition; even applying a weak infusion of opium had limited benefit! Although it began to increase in prevalence in the upper classes in the late nineteenth century, it was almost another century before allergic IgE antibodies were discovered, in 1966, as the underlying mechanism of allergic rhinitis.

'Allergic rhinitis' is the current medical term, which literally means inflammation ('itis') of the nose ('rhino') caused by allergic IgE-mediated reactions. Because this syndrome is often associated with itching and inflammation of the mucous membranes of the eyes (conjunctiva) it is often also referred to as 'allergic rhinoconjunctivitis'.

Just as with other allergic conditions, the symptoms of allergic rhinitis are caused by high levels of IgE directed against allergens; usually to allergens that are inhaled such as pollens, dust mites, animal dander and mould spores. The typical allergic cascade (Chapter 3) is triggered when the allergens bind to IgE on mast cells in the lining of the nose, releasing histamine, leukotrienes and other inflammatory chemicals. Within minutes this causes sneezing, itching, and watering. Chemical mediators released during this immediate or 'acute' reaction also recruit other immune cells which can perpetuate the inflammation and contribute to more 'chronic' symptoms and congestion.

CHANGING PATTERNS OF DISEASE

Although accurate data are not available from one hundred years ago, it is possible that allergic rhinitis was actually one of the first warning signs that industrialisation would eventually lead to an allergy epidemic. Hayfever was certainly becoming more recognised around the early 1900s although it was still far less common than it is today. The eventual rise in asthma, a much more dramatic condition, made the allergic epidemic much more obvious.

The rise in allergic rhinitis has been the most apparent in the last fifty years, particularly in developed nations. An Australian study showed the proportion of adults who experienced hayfever at some point in their lives doubled from 19 per cent in the 1960s to 41 per cent by the 1990s,[4] reflecting similar reports elsewhere.

This also makes allergic rhinitis the most common form of allergic disease. It has the highest rates in adults, but children are also affected. A 1998 report found that 12 per cent of six and seven year olds and almost 20 per cent of thirteen and fourteen year olds had current symptoms of allergic rhinitis.[5] Although the prevalence of asthma has stopped increasing in some regions, the prevalence of allergic rhinitis has continued to increase.[6] Of even greater concern, the number of people affected in highly populated developing countries is also rising significantly.[7]

CONSEQUENCES OF ALLERGIC RHINITIS

Allergic rhinitis affects people in various ways and to varying degrees. In some it is only mild with occasional symptoms, but in others it can be a source of long-standing and major discomfort. When nasal blockage is significant, it can lead to obstructed breathing during sleep ('obstructive sleep apnoea' [OSA]). Periods of reduced oxygen supply can lead to chronic tiredness and problems concentrating during the day. In children, it can affect school performance, behaviour and attention span and can lead to mislabeling with 'attention deficit disorder'. Chronic allergic rhinitis can also be associated with other local problems such as ear infection, hearing problems, sinus infection, nasal polyps and even dental problems due to chronic mouth breathing. Allergic rhinitis is strongly associated with asthma, and in keeping with the 'one airway' concept, uncontrolled inflammation in the upper airways has also been shown to increase the risk of asthma in the lower airways (Chapter 13). Now there is emerging evidence that allergic rhinitis may be associated with other, more generalised effects of systemic inflammation.

IS AIRWAYS INFLAMMATION A SYSTEMIC CONDITION?

Although inflammation is most obvious in the nose (or the chest), there is growing evidence that allergic rhinitis and asthma may have effects much farther afield. One of my Canadian collaborators has elegantly demonstrated that inflammatory products (including cytokines and other mediators, Chapter 5) released from the airways during an allergen challenge circulate through the blood to stimulate immature cells in the bone marrow.[8] This leads to the release of showers of new inflammatory cells that enter the blood stream and come back to sites of inflammation, adding fuel to the fire. It is possible, but not confirmed, that this also contributes to inflammation in blood vessels and increased risk of cardiovascular disease. In support of this idea, higher rates of heart disease have been associated with allergy in both animal and human studies.[9]

Interestingly, treatment of airways inflammation (with inhaled steroids) has also been shown to reduce the risk of heart disease.[10] This highlights the potential for events at a local site to fuel inflammation in other parts of the body, but more research is needed to determine the significance of this.

SIGNS AND SYMPTOMS OF ALLERGIC RHINITIS

In addition to the symptoms of sneezing, congestion, itching (of the eyes and nose), headaches, and morning cough (from post nasal dripping), there are also signs that we can see on physical examination. The dark rings and puffiness under the eyes of some people with allergic rhinitis are called 'allergic shiners'. Patients, especially children, often help us by performing an 'allergic salute' which is doctor-speak for rubbing their nose! This is typically associated with a tell-tale crease across the end of the nose from long-standing frequent upward rubbing. There is also often redness of the eyes sometimes complicated by infective conjunctivitis also from frequent rubbing. When we look in the nose, it is common to see secretions, which are usually clear unless there is a complicating infection. There is often narrowing of the airspace in the nose due to swelling and bogginess of the membranes lining the nose. In children, the adenoids (nose tonsil) may be enlarged adding further to the narrowing. This can also be associated with 'glue ear' (Chapter 10) and hearing difficulties. It is also important to look at other signs of allergic disease such as asthma and eczema.

DIAGNOSING ALLERGIC RHINITIS

The diagnosis is based on the history of symptoms, physical signs and confirmed evidence of allergy on testing. Nasal irritation can have other causes than allergy (including infection, chemical irritants and non-allergic vascular congestion). An important part of taking the history is to obtain information on triggering factors that will help direct the allergy testing. We usually also ask about other illnesses including other allergic conditions in the patient and their family. Information about their home environment and occupation are helpful for understanding possible triggers. We then look for clinical signs of allergic rhinitis and allergic disease (above), followed by allergy skin tests or blood tests (Chapter 10). When asthma is also suspected, lung function testing is also important (Chapter 13). This is especially so in patients with recurrent coughing as it can be hard to distinguish post-nasal drip from asthma. Allergen challenge tests (nasal provocation by inhaling allergens) are available in some centres, mainly for research purposes, but are rarely done routinely. Another important part of any diagnosis is determining the severity and the extent to which it interferes with each patient's quality of life. This has a significant influence of treatment decisions.

CLASSIFYING ALLERGIC RHINITIS

Disease classifications are a useful way of describing severity. There have been several different ways of classifying allergic rhinitis, but the most useful of these is based on the timing of symptoms (intermittent or persistent) and the severity and quality of life (mild, moderate or severe). For example, people with 'persistent' symptoms have been defined as those with symptoms present for more than four days a week, or more than four weeks at a time, in contrast to 'intermittent' symptoms which are present less frequently than this.[11] Those with 'mild' symptoms have no impairment of sleep, daily activities, leisure or sport, school or work, whereas those with 'moderate to severe' disease may have more troublesome symptoms and find that any of all of these activities are affected by their disease.[12] Each person's experience of disease can be different. Even in people who show the same symptoms and signs, some may be extremely bothered by it and others may not.

GENERAL PRINCIPLES OF TREATMENT

As with other allergic conditions, the main aim is to achieve optimal symptom control. This can be done using a combination of strategies including avoiding allergens (if possible) and other triggers and the use of medications. This always depends on the frequency and severity of symptoms.

THE ROLE OF ALLERGEN AVOIDANCE

Reducing exposure to environmental trigger factors is the first approach to consider, especially as this is usually harmless. Although avoidance of some allergens can be difficult, others can be more straight forward (such as avoiding horses if there is a horse allergy). Avoiding allergens such as house dust mite has been controversial because most families cannot achieve the stringent measures that are needed to effectively reduce mite levels. But many practitioners and patients still report benefits using simple strategies, such as bedding covers (where mite level exposure is likely to be greatest). Avoiding pet allergens can also be difficult. Patients are emotionally attached to their pets and often do not want to remove them. If patients are allergic to their pets this is an important consideration, depending on the severity of symptoms. And even if the pet is removed, dander can remain present in the house long after the pet has gone. Pollens can be carried vast distances in the wind, and are very hard to avoid, making pollen immunotherapy the best option for those with significant symptoms.

Avoidance of other non-allergen irritants is also important, such as cigarette smoke and other indoor and outdoor air pollutants.

MEDICATIONS USED IN ALLERGIC RHINITIS

Allergic rhinitis is usually treated with antihistamines and intra-nasal steroid sprays. For mild and intermittent symptoms many patients can achieve symptomatic relief with antihistamine tablets. Antihistamines block histamine receptors to reduce the symptoms caused by histamine release (Chapter 3). They are widely available without a prescription. New generation 'non-sedating' antihistamines are very well tolerated with few side effects. These are preferable to older preparations which can cause drowsiness and significantly impair performance, learning and concentration.

Patients who have more persistent, moderate or severe symptoms are usually prescribed nasal steroid sprays. These are the most effective medications for suppressing the nasal inflammation of allergic rhinitis, and are much more effective that antihistamines. As with asthma, steroid nose sprays need to be used regularly over a period of time in order to achieve their optimal anti-inflammatory benefit. We usually emphasise that symptom control requires long-term treatment for at least a month,[13] although some do feel better much sooner. This is important, because if patients are expecting 'instant relief' they will be disappointed and may discontinue treatment prematurely. If there is no improvement after at least a month, and symptoms are still significant, other options such as immunotherapy need to be considered. This usually requires a specialist referral.

For patients who have allergic rhinoconjunctivitis, antihistamine eye drops are also effective for controlling eye symptoms.

New 'anti-leukotriene' tablets used in asthma may also benefit allergic rhinoconjunctivitis. These work by blocking the action of leukotriene inflammatory products (Chapter 3), but are not as effective as nasal steroids. They appeal to some patients because a single tablet can provide treatment for asthma, allergic rhinitis and allergic rhinoconjunctivitis.

Decongestants do *not* play a role in the long-term management of allergic rhinitis. These medications are available as nasal sprays, tablets and syrups and are mainly used in the short term for viral infections and upper respiratory tract infections. They may be used in special circumstances on a short-term basis in allergic rhinitis (e.g. to help congestion during air travel) but we usually strongly discourage their use in allergic rhinitis.[14] This is because they can make symptoms worse and cause chronic damage to the lining membranes of the nose if used for long periods of time. Patients often suffer from 'rebound congestion' when they stop these medications, and this congestion can be worse than the original symptoms of disease. Similarly, oral steroids are *not* indicated in allergic rhinitis apart from rare cases under specialist supervision. If symptoms are severe enough to warrant this, other long-term treatment options must be considered, such as immunotherapy.

Case Study

Andrew is a nine year old boy who has significant nasal congestion most days. It is worse at night and in the early morning. He snores at night and coughs in the morning. His mother is annoyed by his constant sniffing. He is tired during the day, not concentrating at school and his teacher is concerned about his progress and his behaviour in the classroom. His eyes are often red and itchy. His mother first tried using an over-the-counter antihistamine but this made him even drowsier. Their pharmacist advised using a non-sedating antihistamine which only partially improved Andrew's symptoms. His family doctor referred him to our clinic for allergy testing, which was positive to house dust mites but no other major allergens. He had an overnight sleep study which did not show any significant sleep apnoea (obstructive breathing). He had lung function testing, with signs of mild reduction in airflow which responded to bronchodilators. His parents were advised to consider covering his pillows, mattress and quilt with dust mite proof covers, and he was started on a daily steroid nasal spray and antihistamine eye drops. He was also prescribed an asthma bronchodilator (Chapter 13) for use if he experiences coughing and chest tightness. When he was reviewed three months later all his symptoms and his lung function were significantly better. He has had no side effects from the nose spray. We reviewed him again one year later and he had some persistent nasal symptoms. The option of immunotherapy was discussed, but Andrew was reluctant and the family has opted to wait and see how he goes. They would prefer to continue symptomatic treatment knowing that immunotherapy may be a viable option in the future. If it does become necessary, Andrew has said that he would prefer to try the sublingual immune therapy (SLIT) rather than injection immunotherapy (Chapter 10).

POINTS THIS CASE ILLUSTRATES

- Andrew has persistent allergic rhinoconjunctivitis with moderate symptoms. This is unlikely to respond to antihistamines alone
- Allergic rhinitis allergic rhinitis can present as learning and behavioural problems in children
- Sedating antihistamines should be avoided as they also cause drowsiness and poor performance. Non-sedating antihistamines are helpful but not as effective as nasal steroids
- Nasal obstruction can cause obstructed breathing and choking at night, although this was not the case in Andrew. Overnight sleep monitoring is useful to determine if there is 'obstructive sleep apnoea'
- Allergic rhinitis is often associated with asthma. Andrew's morning cough could be due to postnasal drip or asthma, and lung function tests were useful to make this distinction
- Using the nasal steroid may have been a factor in improving Andrew's lung function
- Andrew showed a fairly good response to simple measures but it is difficult to say if this was due to the allergen avoidance or the nasal steroids (or both)
- Immunotherapy could be a useful treatment option for Andrew in the future particularly if his symptoms persist. The preferences of the family and/or the patient play a major role in this decision

- Sublingual immunotherapy is often the preferred form of immuno-therapy in children (but is not available in some centres).

SAFETY OF INTRANASAL STEROID SPRAYS

Nasal steroid sprays are very safe and well tolerated in both adults and children. They can be used long term without damage to the lining of the nose. Some people experience local irritation and dry-ness but this can be reduced by saline drops. There is no evidence that these medications have any of the side effects associated with oral steroids.[15] Newer generation of nasal steroids have also been designed so their absorption is minimal when they are swallowed with nasal secretions. These medications are also the treatment of choice in children with allergic rhinitis, and follow-up studies have shown no evidence of effects on growth.[16] However, if inhaled steroids are also being used for asthma in the same patient, the total daily dose (delivered to the nose and the chest) needs to be considered and minimised where possible (Chapter 13).

THE UNITED AIRWAYS

As previously discussed (Chapter 13) the associations between aller-gic rhinitis and asthma is important. Patients with allergic rhinitis may have mild asthma without realising it, so it is important that we check for this. Similarly, people with asthma may have sinus inflammation without realising it and this untreated inflamma-tion in the upper airways can exacerbate their asthma symptoms. Effective treatment of allergic rhinitis with nasal steroids have been shown to also improve asthma.

THE NATURAL HISTORY OF ALLERGIC RHINITIS: WHAT HAPPENS WITH AGE

Allergic rhinitis often begins in childhood, and the 'atopic' state (IgE production) typically persists well into adult life, although symptoms will vary from year to year. Some have later onset and allergic rhinitis is generally most common between the ages of twenty-five and forty-four.[17] Unlike sensitisation to foods, which can disappear with age, once sensitisation to inhaled allergens is established, it rarely goes away. This is why diseases that are induced by inhaled allergens also tend to persist with age. Some people naturally experience an improvement with symptoms over time, but even then allergy tests are likely to stay positive.

THE ROLE OF IMMUNOTHERAPY IN ALLERGIC RHINITIS

Currently, immunotherapy is the only potential curative treatment for allergic disease. There is very strong evidence that immuno-therapy (Chapter 10) can be effective in the treatment of allergic rhinitis and allergic rhinoconjunctivitis. Unlike other medications, immunotherapy targets and suppresses the underlying Type 2 allergic immune response (Chapter 5). By addressing the immune problem that causes allergies it is the only treatment that can alter the natural history of disease.

This is a very good treatment option in patients who have moderate, severe or persistent disease who still have symptoms after trying symptomatic treatments. Immunotherapy is avail-able for most common inhaled allergens and has proven benefits in patients sensitised to house dust mite, grass and tree pollens, moulds and some animal danders. There are regional differences in the most prevalent allergens, with many different products and different immunotherapy regimes around the world. But the basic principles are the same – an up-dosing schedule followed by a maintenance period (of several years) with appropriate precautions for potential allergen reactions (Chapter 10). Immunotherapy for allergic rhinitis can be beneficial for asthma and even eczema in the same patient. There is also preliminary evidence that early use may reduce disease progression from allergic rhinitis to asthma and reduce the development of new sensitisations. Although immu-notherapy has been traditionally given by injection, recent studies have shown that high dose allergen tablets/drops placed under the tongue (sublingual immunotherapy) can also be effective, which is a more attractive option for many patients, particularly children (Chapter 10).

• • •

Allergic rhinoconjunctivitis is one of the most common conditions affecting adults and children in urbanised communities, and it is far from being a trivial condition. It can have substantial personal, social and economic costs. Significant advances in immunotherapy have provided curative treatment in many, but not all, patients. There are many new developments afoot that are aimed at making immunotherapy more effective and safer with more convenient dosing and delivery methods.

15

Other assorted allergies

It is theoretically possible to be allergic to almost any potential allergen, and impossible to cover every possible scenario. But there are some other common conditions that we see regularly in our clinics that are certainly worth a mention here.

INSECT ALLERGY

Allergic reactions to insect stings is another common reason for referral in both adults and children. These patients typically present with a typical acute IgE-mediated allergic reaction (Chapter 3) usually within minutes to an hour after a sting, typically from honey bees, wasps or (in southern Australia) to jack jumper ants.

The range of reactions varies from a large local reaction, through to a mild generalised reaction (rash but no anaphylaxis) to a serious generalised reaction (anaphylaxis). These patients need immediate management of their reaction with emergency adrenaline treatment if there is evidence of anaphylaxis.

Once the reaction has settled, it is important that they are discharged from the emergency centre with an adrenaline auto-injector and an 'anaphylaxis action plan' in the event of another sting. They also need to be referred for specialist assessments, particularly if there have been any generalised symptoms. This is so that allergic testing can be performed to confirm the insect allergy and to determine whether insect venom immunotherapy is indicated. Allergy testing is usually delayed for at least four weeks after a sting as consumption of the IgE during a reaction can lead to a false negative test.

Adults with confirmed allergy tests who have had any systemic reactions (anaphylactic or not) are recommended to commence immunotherapy. This is because the risk of serious anaphylaxis to future stings is highest in adults. The threshold for treatment in young children is slightly higher, and immunotherapy is usually reserved for those who have had symptoms suggestive of anaphylaxis.

Immunotherapy is highly effective and usually curative in patients with insect allergies (such as bee venom allergy). Once patients have been on maintenance doses of immunotherapy for at least six months they usually no longer need to carry their adrenaline auto-injectors, apart from when they are likely to be in remote areas away from medical access. At the completion of the immunotherapy (usually several years depending on the protocol used) we can usually confidently say that the risk of future anaphylaxis is reduced significantly to only slightly above the risk of the normal population. Only a very small proportion of patients does not respond as well and need to continue immunotherapy for longer periods of time.

Drug and latex allergies

Most reactions to therapeutic drugs are not due to allergy. Less than one in ten drug reactions are actually due to an immune reaction. These can be either due to an IgE reaction with typical acute 'IgE symptoms' within an hour (Chapter 3) or cell mediated skin reactions and other symptoms such as fever and joint pains which are delayed more than an hour.[1] The history and evaluation of the reaction are very important for making the diagnosis, because allergy testing is only available in a select few cases. It is important to know the relationship between the drug and the symptoms, the severity and nature of the symptoms, and the time course of the symptoms after the reactions.

Reactions to antibiotics are one of the most common reported drug reactions, but many of these patients are not actually allergic. Rashes are very common with viral infections, especially in children, and may be unrelated to antibiotics that happen to have been prescribed (perhaps unnecessarily). We therefore quite frequently see children who have been mislabelled as allergic to penicillin for many years. In many cases the probability of allergy is so low we may proceed directly to an oral challenge with the antibiotics to show that the patient is not allergic. For penicillin and some other antibiotics we are able to perform IgE allergy tests (blood tests and skin tests). This is useful if the history is less certain. A positive blood test is a good indication of allergy and the drug is best avoided. If the blood test is negative this does not exclude an allergy and we usually proceed to do a series of skin tests (superficial and then deeper) which are more sensitive. If these are still negative, an allergy is very unlikely and we usually proceed to an antibiotic challenge to prove there is no current allergy. We always stress to patients that a negative allergy testing/ challenge mean that they are not allergic *now*, but it does not exclude a new allergy developing at some point in the future.

For many other drugs, there are no allergy tests available, and challenges are the only definitive way of confirming reactions. However, because some reactions can be very severe and life threatening, drug challenges are not usually undertaken unless the previous reaction was mild or moderate, or the likelihood of allergy is low. When the probability of allergy is high and the previous symptoms were severe, we usually deem the risk of a challenge too high to recommend that the drug is completely avoided. In most cases, alternative unrelated drugs are available. Most countries have a medical-alert system and bracelets or medallions are issued to indicate the drug allergy warning.

In rare instances when patients have a serious condition that requires treatment and there is no other viable alternative, a rapid desensitisation procedure can be performed. This is dangerous and must be done under specialist care. It involves starting with very low doses of the drug and giving relatively rapid increases of the drug over a short period (usually hours) to achieve the full therapeutic dose. Reactions during the desenstisation procedure are treated, but the up-dosing still continues despite the reaction because the drug is considered essential. If the drug is needed for an extended period, it must continue to be given daily to maintain the desensitised state. If it is discontinued, the patient will need to go through the same procedure in the future if the drug is ever needed again.

Latex (rubber) is another common allergen, which can cause symptoms ranging from localised itching and contact dermatitis through to anaphylaxis in sensitised patients. The diagnosis is suspected when symptoms occur on contact with products made of latex, such as balloons, condoms and surgical gloves. Allergy tests are available for latex to confirm the diagnosis (by blood test, skin test and challenge tests). Many latex allergic patients are also allergic to certain stone fruits (so it is important to look for latex allergy in these conditions and vice versa). Avoidance is the best approach, with an appropriate action plan in the event of accidental exposure. It is particularly important to document latex allergy in patients having dental or surgical procedures, so that latex-free gloves and a latex-free theatre environment can be arranged to avoid anaphylaxis during the procedure when the patient may be anaesthetised.

Papular urticaria (skin reactions to insect bites)

This is one of the most common forms of hives, especially in children, and appears as groups of itchy, lumpy welts or lumps, usually in areas of exposed skin. It is due to a localised immune reaction to the saliva of biting insects, most commonly mosquitoes, fleas and lice. Unlike other hives, these lesions can persist for many days. It is most common in young school age children and improves with age, as tolerance occurs after repeated exposure. Reactions are rarely serious and anaphylaxis is very rare. Antihistamines are useful to treat the itching during episodes but it is best managed by reducing exposure to the insects, by using insect repellants and by removing animals that may carry insects (cats, dogs, and pet birds). Sometimes treatment for secondary bacterial infection is necessary.

'Allergic' reactions to exercise, water, cold, heat and other physical factors (physical urticarias)

The 'allergic' reactions that seem to surprise people the most are reactions to physical factors, including exercise, cold temperatures, heat, physical pressure, vibration, sun and even plain water! Although the underlying processes are not completely clear, these physical factors seem to be caused by the release of histamines, leukotrienes and other mediators of the allergic response from the mast cells (Chapter 3) in the skin. In other words, these reactions are not caused by the IgE allergic antibodies but by direct physical release of allergic mediators. Luckily, individual patients generally react to just of one of these triggers, rather than to all of them.

These conditions range in severity from itchy transient skin lesions, to potential anaphylactic reactions. Fortunately, the severe forms are rare, but can be seen in some patients with exercise-induced symptoms and some cases of cold-induced urticaria when there is whole body exposure (such as swimming in cold water). In one unusual form of exercise-induced anaphylaxis, the reaction is food-dependent and *only* occurs when exercise occurs after eating the food (but curiously not when food or exercise is undertaken separately).

The diagnosis is usually suspected based on the history and confirmed with a challenge to the suspected physical agent, such as placing an ice block on the forearm (for cold urticaria), an exercise test, applying pressure, heat, light, water and so on. The treatment is usually a combination of avoiding or minimising exposure to the triggering agent and using antihistamines when this is not completely possible. The rare patients with anaphylactic symptoms also need to carry adrenalin auto-injectors.

PERSISTENT HIVES WITH NO APPARENT CAUSE: CHRONIC IDIOPATHIC URTICARIA (CIU)

Transient hives (urticaria) are very common and probably affect one in four people at some stage in their lives.[2] However, in a small group of people urticaria is recurring and long standing. In this context the definition of 'chronic' requires that the urticaria has been present for more than six weeks, but in some patients this goes on for months or even years. While some have a clear triggering factor (above) most have no apparent cause, and earn the label 'idiopathic' which is a term we often use when we really have no idea!

But CIU is a diagnosis of exclusion, when other underlying causes of urticaria have been excluded such as infection, hidden food allergies and autoimmune disease. Although some studies have suggested a link between *Helicobacter pylori* (the bacteria that is associated with stomach ulcers) and chronic urticaria, this has not been proven. Some doctors still look for this and other intestinal infestations in patients with unexplained urticaria.

In most patients no cause is found and the mechanism is unclear. Some studies suggest that CIU may happen when the immune system makes non-allergic IgG antibodies to the patient's own IgE receptors, thus triggering the histamine cascade.[3] One way of assessing this is to take the patient's own serum (containing the IgG antibodies) and applying this as a skin test by injecting it back under their skin. In patients with CIU it is common to see a positive test reaction to their own serum. I have seen this many times, but we don't usually do it routinely. It is a good way of showing that the patient is reacting to themselves, and makes other causes unlikely. But the treatment is ultimately the same.

Symptomatic control is the main aim of treatment. This condition may not be serious but it can be extremely itchy, unsightly and embarrassing. Because it can last for many months, patients often become quite miserable. Regular antihistamines are the main treatment used. In some patients the addition of a second drug may be needed to control symptoms. Normal antihistamines used in allergy block Type 1 histamine receptors, but there is another group of drugs (used routinely to treat gastric ulcers and stomach acid related disease) which actually work by blocking Type 2 histamine receptors. A combination of these treatments can be effective in many CIU patients. Leukotriene inhibitors have also been tried in CIU although their role has not been confirmed. Earlier strategies such as exclusion diets (to remove food additives and preservatives) have also not been proven to be effective, probably because food additives are a very uncommon cause of chronic urticaria. Although it can take a long time, this condition usually eventually burns itself out, with only about 20 per cent of patients with CIU still having symptoms after one year.[4]

16

Where to from here?

As we arrive at the end of this particular journey, it is clear that we are really on the threshold of another. We can see how the challenges facing our immune systems have changed so dramatically over the last fifty years. So much about our world has changed since, as a young doctor in the 1930s, my grandmother Monica first saw the immune system rescued from its battle against serious bacterial threats. Her main work was with women's and infant's health, at a time when antibiotics made the difference between life and death for many new mothers and their newborn babies. Now we face new challenges, as we become increasingly prone to pointless, misdirected reactions to common harmless things in the environment, and even our own body tissues; all the result of modern environmental changes. Ironically it is that victory over the microbial world that might have led us to this new epidemic of allergic disease. But there is probably more to it than that. And although allergic diseases are a major part of this story, the problem is so much bigger. Now one of the greatest challenges of modern medicine is to learn how we can live in the new world we have created. To restore a form of immune balance so that we are less prone to the growing number of modern diseases that result from varying kinds of inflammation or immune failure.

It is becoming increasingly unlikely that allergies and immune diseases are due to specific gene defects, but rather due to *shifts in patterns* of gene expression in intricate immune networks. These shifts in immune function are being driven by environmental changes, which are complex and still not well defined. But it *is* clear that these effects begin in pregnancy when the developing immune system is most sensitive to change, and continue to have an influence in the early years after birth. Different factors are likely to have different effects, depending on our age. To solve this problem it is critical that we promote research into early life events as a future priority. This will provide new insights into how diseases develop, what factors drive this, and how these can be prevented more effectively. Greater understanding of individual differences in genetic susceptibility will help us predict disease more accurately, and lead to more individualised strategies for treatment and prevention.

At this stage, the complexity of the genetic and environmental interactions is overwhelming, but the development of new research approaches, mathematical modelling and network theory, will provide us with greater capacity to study these complex interactions.

While these goals are futuristic and seem more in the realms of science fiction, it is important that we try to hold a broad vision and avoid narrowing our ideas. The phenomenal scientific progress in the last hundred years, gives us great hope for the future. As always we need an open mind; ready to embrace the new discoveries, new solutions and new ways of thinking.

• • •

For myself, this journey of immunological adventures has provided many new reflections. I have a renewed appreciation for just how far we have come. Our focus in medicine is naturally on what we don't know – so that we can work to expand our frontiers of knowledge. But the danger of always looking into the vast abyss of the unknown, is that it can leave us feeling tiny, holding our current bag of knowledge, so small compared to what is still to come. We always seem to be apologising for not having the answers and often feel we are letting our patients down. But now I am reminded that, while there are still many questions, we have learned so much about the immune system, which lay almost completely undiscovered one hundred years ago. We have seen many completely new fields of science and medicine develop, even if we only look at the last ten years. We have much better treatments than ever before. And all of this is growing at an exponential rate as our technologies and computing capacity continue to expand beyond anything that we could have imagined when the story of these modern diseases began.

When I started my journey into medicine, inspired by Monica's stories and adventures I had no way of knowing where it would lead me. Then our current predicament had not yet come fully into focus. Although the signs of a changing disease profile were emerging, we had not yet put it together. Monica had always strongly believed that promoting women's and infant's health was the key to improving societal health and well-being, long before the 'fetal origins' hypothesis was formally born. So it now takes great personal meaning to find myself also working in the same field, although the landscape might be unrecognisable from what she once saw.

Monica had been my inspiration to study medicine, so when I was asked to give the keynote address at the Centenary Women's Trust annual luncheon a few years ago, describing my own career and achievements, I thought instead that I would honour hers. It was 2007, the fiftieth anniversary of our Medical School and I was also there to tell the story of my grandfather Sir Stanley and his role as the founding Vice Chancellor. But as it was an occasion to celebrate the academic development of women, I decided instead to tell their story from my grandmother Monica's perspective. She had been a strong influence throughout my career. Monica had just turned ninety-four at that time, and was absolutely thrilled that I was invited to give such an important public address. She was so excited and looking forward to being there too. The Governor General of Australia and many other dignitaries were present, and so many people who had known Monica and Stanley. Sadly the occasion was made ever so much more meaningful by her death only just a few short weeks before. Difficult as it was for me to tell her story through my grief, there could not have been a more fitting way to celebrate her life. Although her chair was empty, I could feel her and Stanley there in spirit. I was quite overwhelmed by the response. People were so touched and so impressed that a woman born into poverty in 1913 could have quietly achieved so much with just a positive attitude and without apparent concern for prevailing belief systems that might have curtailed a woman's ambitions. Most importantly, it was an opportunity to share her philosophies, which also shaped my life so much. That we should always look for the good in every situation. That we should never stop having fun. And that 'where there is a will, there is a way', her life-long motto which embodied much of who she was, and had a great influence on my approach and personal philosophies.

And of course, I think back to why I 'put pen to paper' here in the first place; to share our knowledge, theories and uncertainties. As we learn more about the immune system, allergies and our current predicament we need to share it, not just with our medical and scientific colleagues but with the many people that are affected in some way. I think of all the many questions that our patients and their families have every day. And the theories. We have learned a lot and we still have a lot more to learn yet. Sometimes the biggest steps forward come from people thinking completely 'outside the box'. People from another field altogether, with a different vantage point, untainted by the dogma we have created to make sense of complexity. We need to be open to new ideas. New approaches. But we also need to find solutions that will not create more problems. Strong scientific rigor is needed to continue to pursue new approaches as they arise, as well as the many existing avenues of investigation. This is a global problem and a global effort to combat this is now well underway. All this will take time, but there is cause for great optimism and anticipation. I hope that it will not be too long before we can provide another installment with a few more answers! This is a very exciting time and I can't wait to see what happens next.

ACKNOWLEDGMENTS

My journey into the mystery of allergic diseases began over twenty years ago, and there are so many people who have provided encouragement, guidance and inspiration along the way. The main inspiration to study medicine came from grandmother Monica. One of few women doctors in her time, she was driven by a desire to help the underprivileged, especially women and children. It was my grandfather Sir Stanley Prescott who instilled my interest in medical research and education, and I am ever grateful to Professor Lawrie Beilin who gave me my first wonderful taste of clinical research. My deepest thanks also to Professor Fiona Stanley, who has been cheering me on from the sidelines since I started my career. A woman in medicine could not have a more inspiring role model. Thank you Fiona for believing in me and helping me see my own potential. It was Professor Patrick Holt who first drew me into the world of the immune system with his incredible and intelligent insights. I thank him for the chance to work in his laboratory and get hands-on experience at the 'bench'. After finishing my PhD, I had to 'go it alone' and set up my own clinical research team and my own lab, and this would not have been possible without the support of my first PhD students Jan Dunstan, Angie Taylor and Paul Noakes. They are all so wonderful and I have so many happy memories of the early days of our group. Their dedication and commitment inspired the PhD students who followed including Liza Breckler, David Martino, Suzanne Meldrum, Nina D'Vaz and all of the new students we have today. We are all so grateful to the many research assistants and research nurses who have worked on our research projects over the years. I also thank Professors Meri Tulic and Debbie Palmer who joined my team more recently to help me in the leadership of a steadily growing team. Of course, my deepest thanks also goes to the families and the children who have participated in our research studies. Without the help and support of our community, none of our efforts would be possible.

Many of us like to think we have 'a book waiting inside of us', and I want to thank Professor Terri-ann White at UWA Publishing for helping me find mine. It was her vision that made this a reality. Thank you for believing in this. And to Anne Ryden who was always encouraging, enthusiastic and patient as we assembled this work.

I would particularly like to thank Professor Ruby Pawankar, President-elect of the World Allergy Organization, for writing the foreword. An inspiring international leader, Ruby is dedicated to improving knowledge and understanding of allergic diseases, and always aims for better care and prevention of these conditions. She is a wonderful and generous person and I am very greateful for her support in this endeavour.

Dearest of all, my husband Craig, whose love and support means more than any words can say. Thank you for your perspectives, your encouragement, and particularly your patience and understanding as I devoted my energy to this other passion. To my parents, thank you for teaching me always to look for the higher purpose in everything I do, something Craig makes sure I never forget.

Finally, to the families who attend our clinic suffering from many kinds of allergic and immune diseases, it was your experiences, your struggles, your questions, thoughts and ideas that inspired me to write this. You are the reason for this, and this is all for you.

NOTES

Chapter 3 — In the classroom: some basics of allergy

1   C. Agostoni, et al., 'Complementary feeding: a commentary by the ESPGHAN Committee on Nutrition'; F. R. Greer, et al., 'Effects of early nutritional interventions on the development of atopic disease in infants and children: the role of maternal dietary restriction, breastfeeding, timing of introduction of complementary foods, and hydrolyzed formulas; A. Host, et al., 'Dietary prevention of allergic diseases in infants and small children'; S. L. Prescott, et al., 'The importance of early complementary feeding in the development of oral tolerance: concerns and controversies'.

2   Infant Feeding Advice, Australasian Society of Allergy and Immunology.

Chapter 4 — On the world stage: a global perspective

1   This figure shows the time-trends for each disease over the last fifty–sixty years. It shows the proportional increase, not actual levels, and is based on data from various sources (including Armitage 2001, Gale 2002, Ninan 1992, Aberg 1995, Carr 1964, Nakagomi 1994, Peat 1994, Mullins 2007, Danchenko 2006) and on concepts of Bach 2002.

2   H. Renz, et al., 'Gene-environment interactions in chronic inflammatory disease'.

3   M. I. Asher, et al., 'Worldwide time trends in the prevalence of symptoms of asthma, allergic rhinoconjunctivitis, and eczema in childhood'.

4   same as above.; C. K. Lai, et al., 'Global variation in the prevalence and severity of asthma symptoms'; N. Ait-Khaled, et al., 'Global map of the prevalence of symptoms of rhinoconjunctivitis in children'; J. A. Odhiambo, et al., 'Global map of eczema'.

5   O. C. Herbert, et al., 'Western lifestyle and increased prevalence of atopic diseases'.

6   J. Peat, et al., 'Changing prevalence of asthma in Australian school children'.

7   J. L. Hopper, et al., 'Increase in the self-reported prevalence of asthma and hay fever in adults over the last generation: a matched parent-offspring study'.

8   M. I. Asher, et al., 'Worldwide time trends'; C. F. Robertson, et al., 'Asthma prevalence in Melbourne schoolchildren: have we reached the peak?'.

9   R. J. Mullins, 'Paediatric food allergy trends in a community-based specialist allergy practice, 1995–2006'; S. H. Sicherer, et al., 'US prevalence of self-reported peanut, tree nut, and sesame allergy: 11-year follow-up'.

10   C. Venter, et al., 'Prevalence of sensitization reported and objectively assessed food hypersensitivity amongst six-year-old children: a population-based study'; M. Osterballe, et al., 'The prevalence of food hypersensitivity in an unselected population of children and adults'; S. H. Sicherer and H. A. Sampson, 'Food allergy'.

11   E. Ostblom, et al., 'Reported symptoms of food hypersensitivity and sensitization to common foods in 4-year-old children'.

12   R. J. Mullins, 'Paediatric food allergy trends'.

13   A. Soni, 'Allergic rhinitis: trends in use and expenditures', 2000 and 2005, Medical Expenditure Panel Survey.

14   same as above.

15   same as above.

16   S. L. Prescott and K. A. Allen, 'Food Allergy: Riding the second wave of the allergy epidemic'.

17   For a review paper that covers this, see S. L. Prescott and K. A. Allen, 'Food Allergy'.

18   N. J. Osborne, et al., 'Prevalence of challenge-proven IgE-mediated food allergy using population-based sampling and predetermined challenge criteria in infants'.

19   R. J. Mullins, 'Paediatric food allergy trends '.

Chapter 5 — Down the rabbit hole: into the immune system

1   T. R. Mosmann and R. L. Coffman, 'Heterogeneity of cytokine secretion patterns and functions of helper T cells'.

2   G. Lack, 'Epidemiologic risks for food allergy'.

3   P. Varshney, et al., 'A randomized controlled study of peanut oral immunotherapy: clinical desensitization and modulation of the allergic response'.

4   J. F. Bach, 'The effect of infections on susceptibility to autoimmune and allergic diseases'.

5   same as above.

6   M. Wills-Karp, J. Santeliz and C. L. Karp, 'The germless theory of allergic disease: revisiting the hygiene hypothesis'.

7   same as above; and J. F. Bach, 'The effect of infections on susceptibility to autoimmune and allergic diseases'.

8   C. L. Bennett, et al., 'The immune dysregulation, polyendocrinopathy, enteropathy, X-linked syndrome (IPEX) is caused by mutations of FOXP3'.

9   same as above.

Chapter 6 — Setting the scene: the importance of early life

1   D. J. Barker, 'Fetal origins of coronary heart disease'.

2   M. Hanson and P. Gluckman, 'Developmental origins of noncommunicable disease: population and public health implications'.

3   P. D. Wadhwa, et al., 'Developmental origins of health and disease: brief history of the approach and current focus on epigenetic mechanisms'.

4   D. Barker et al., 'Weight in infancy and death from ischemic heart disease'.

5   S. J. Simpson and G. A. Sword, 'Phase polyphenism in locusts: Mechanisms, population consequences, adaptive significance and evolution'.

6   T. G. Wegmann et al., 'Bidirectional cytokine interactions in the maternal-fetal relationship: is successful pregnancy a Th2 phenomenon?'

7   L. A. Breckler, et al., 'Modulation of in vivo and in vitro cytokine production over the course of pregnancy in allergic and non-allergic mothers'.

8   V. R. Aluvihare, M. Kallikourdis and A. G. Betz, 'Regulatory T cells mediate maternal tolerance to the fetus'.

9   S. Prescott, et al., 'Transplacental priming of the human immune system to environmental allergens: universal skewing of initial T-cell responses towards Th-2 cytokine profile'; S. Prescott, 'Development of allergen-specific T-cell memory in atopic and normal children'.

10   S. L. Prescott, et al., 'Transplacental priming of the human immune system'.

11   S. L. Prescott, et al., 'Development of allergen-specific T-cell memory'.

12   same as above.

13   D. P. Strachan, 'Hay fever, hygiene, and household size'; D. P. Strachan, 'Family size, infection and atopy: the first decade of the

"hygiene hypothesis"'.

14 M. L. K. Tang, et al., 'Reduced interferon gamma secretion in neonates and subsequent atopy'; S. L. Prescott, et al., 'Reciprocal age-related patterns of allergen-specific T-cell immunity in normal vs. atopic infants', discussion pp. 50–1; S. L. Prescott and P.G. Holt, 'Abnormalities in cord blood mononuclear cytokine production as a predictor of later atopic disease in childhood'.

15 S. L. Prescott, et al., 'Development of allergen-specific T-cell memory'.

16 M. Tulic, et al., 'Differences in the developmental trajectory of innate microbial responses in atopic and normal children: new insights into immune ontogeny'.

17 S. L. Prescott, et al., 'Protein kinase-C zeta: a novel "protective" neonatal T cell marker that can be up-regulated by allergy prevention strategies'.

18 same as above.

19 N. D'Vaz, et al., 'Neonatal T cell protein kinase C zeta as a screening test for predicting allergic disease and disease severity'.

20 M. Tulic, et al., 'Differences in the developmental trajectory of innate microbial responses'.

21 S. L. Prescott, et al., 'Development of allergen-specific T-cell memory'.

22 M. Tulic, et al., 'Differences in the developmental trajectory of innate microbial responses'.

23 P. Amoudruz, 'Impaired Toll-like receptor 2 signalling in monocytes from 5-year-old allergic children'.

24 M. Smith, et al., 'Children with egg allergy have evidence of reduced neonatal CD4(+)CD25(+)CD127(lo/-) regulatory T cell function'; B. Schaub, et al., 'Impairment of T-regulatory cells in cord blood of atopic mothers'; B. Schaub, et al., 'Maternal farm exposure modulates neonatal immune mechanisms through regulatory T cells'.

25 D. Martino and S. L. Prescott, 'Silent mysteries: epigenetic paradigms could hold the key to conquering the epidemic of allergy and immune disease'.

26 B. Schaub, et al., 'Maternal farm exposure'.

27 S. L. Prescott and V. L. Clifton, 'Asthma and Pregnancy: emerging evidence of epigenetic interactions in utero'.

28 N. Sudo, et al., 'The requirement of intestinal bacterial flora for the development of an IgE production system fully susceptible to oral tolerance induction'.

29 E. Sepp, et al., 'Intestinal microflora of Estonian and Swedish infants'.

30 same as above.

31 B. Björkstén, et al, 'Allergy development and the intestinal microflora during the first year of life'; M. Kalliomäki, et al., 'Distinct patterns

of neonatal gut microflora in infants in whom atopy was and was not developing'; Y. M. Sjogren, et al., 'Altered early infant gut microbiota in children developing allergy up to 5 years of age'.

32 M. Kalliomäki, et al., 'Distinct patterns of neonatal gut microflora in infants in whom atopy was and was not developing'; B. Björkstén, et al., 'Allergy development and the intestinal microflora during the first year of life'.

33 M. F. Bottcher, et al., 'Microflora-associated characteristics in faeces from allergic and nonallergic infants'.

34 B. Björkstén, et al., 'The intestinal microflora in allergic Estonian and Swedish 2-year-old children'.

35 Y. M. Sjogren, et al., 'Altered early infant gut microbiota in children developing allergy up to 5 years of age'.

36 S. L. Prescott and B. Björkstén, 'Probiotics for the prevention or treatment of allergic diseases'.

37 same as above.

Chapter 7 — Genetics and allergic disease

1   N. I. Kjellman, 'Prediction and prevention of atopic allergy'; R. S. Zeiger, et al., 'Genetic and environmental factors affecting the development of atopy through age 4 in children with atopic parents: a prospective radomised study of food allergen avoidance'.

2   W. Cookson, et al., 'Linkage between Immunoglobulin E responses underlying asthma and rhinitis and chromosome 11q'.

3   same as above.

4   M. Baldini, et al., 'A Polymorphism in the 5' flanking region of the CD14 gene is associated with circulating soluble CD14 levels and with total serum immunoglobulin E'; P. S. Gao, et al., 'Serum total IgE levels and CD14 on chromosome 5q31'.

5   Figure 11 is an illustration of the concept based on existing studies rather than actual data. Information to draw this figure was taken from M. Baldini, et al., 'A Polymorphism in the 5' flanking region of the CD14 gene'; P. S. Gao, et al., 'Serum total IgE levels and CD14 on chromosome 5q31'; G. H. Koppelman, et al., 'Association of a promoter polymorphism of the CD14 gene and atopy'; and T. F. Leung, et al., 'The C–159T polymorphism in the CD14 promoter is associated with serum total IgE concentration in atopic Chinese children'.

6   G. H. Koppelman, et al., 'Association of a promoter polymorphism'; T. F. Leung, et al., 'The C–159T polymorphism in the CD14 promoter'.

7   Figure 12 is an illustration of the concept based on existing studies

rather than the actual data. Information to draw this figure was taken from C. Ober, et al., 'A second-generation genome-wide screen for asthma-susceptibility alleles in a founder population'; W. Eder, et al., 'Opposite effects of CD 14/-260 on serum IgE levels in children raised in different environments'; and A. Simpson, et al., 'Endotoxin exposure, CD14, and allergic disease: an interaction between genes and the environment'.

8   C. Ober, et al., 'A second-generation genome-wide screen'.
9   Figure 13 is an illustration of the concept based on existing studies rather than actual data. Information to draw this figure was taken from W. Eder, et al., 'Opposite effects of CD 14/-260'; and A. Simpson, et al., 'Endotoxin exposure'.
10   W. Eder et al., 'Opposite effects of CD 14/-260'; A. Simpson, et al., 'Endotoxin exposure, CD14, and allergic disease: an interaction between genes and the environment'.

Chapter 8 — The environmental suspects in the allergy epidemic

1   E. von Mutius, et al., 'Prevalence of asthma and atopy in two areas of West and East Germany'.
2   E. von Mutius, et al., 'Increasing prevalence of hay fever and atopy among children in Leipzig, East Germany'.
3   D. P. Strachan, 'Family size, infection and atopy: the first decade of the "hygiene hypothesis"'.
4   S. L. Prescott, 'Allergy: the price we pay for cleaner living?'.
5   J. F. Bach, 'The effect of infections on susceptibility to autoimmune and allergic diseases'.
6   B. Björkstén, 'The gut microbiota: a complex ecosystem'.
7   N. Sudo, et al., 'The requirement of intestinal bacterial flora for the development of an IgE production system fully susceptible to oral tolerance induction'.
8   Y. M. Sjogren, et al., 'Altered early infant gut microbiota in children developing allergy up to 5 years of age'.
9   N. Blumer, et al., 'Perinatal maternal application of *Lactobacillus rhamnosus* GG suppresses allergic airway inflammation in mouse offspring'; N. Blumer, et al., 'Prenatal lipopolysaccharide-exposure prevents allergic sensitisation and airway inflammation, but not airway responsiveness in a murine model of experimental asthma'.
10   W. H. Oddy, et al., 'The effects of respiratory infections, atopy, and breastfeeding on childhood asthma'.
11   P. G. Holt and P.D. Sly, 'Interactions between respiratory tract infections and atopy in the aetiology of asthma'.

12 N. Sigurs, et al., 'Asthma and immunoglobulin E antibodies after respiratory syncytial virus bronchiolitis: a prospective cohort study with matched controls'.

13 J. Rowe, et al., 'Heterogeneity in diphtheria-tetanus-acellular pertussis vaccine – specific cellular immunity during infancy: relationship to variations in the kinetics of postnatal maturation of systemic th1 function'.

14 P. G. Holt and P. D. Sly, 'Interactions between respiratory tract infections and atopy'; J. Rowe, et al., 'Heterogeneity in diphtheria-tetanus-acellular pertussis vaccine-specific cellular immunity during infancy'.

15 R. J. Mullins and C. A. Camargo Jr., 'Shining a light on vitamin D and its impact on the developing immune system'; S. T. Weiss and A. A. Litonjua, 'The in utero effects of maternal vitamin D deficiency: How it results in asthma and other chronic diseases'.

16 B. A. Raby, et al., 'Association of vitamin D receptor gene polymorphisms with childhood and adult asthma'.

17 S. T. Weiss, 'Bacterial components plus vitamin D: The ultimate solution to the asthma (autoimmune disease) epidemic?'.

18 C. A. Camargo, et al., 'Regional differences in EpiPen prescriptions in the United States: the potential role of vitamin D'.

19 M. F. Vassallo, et al., 'Season of birth and food allergy in children.'

20 R. J. Mullins, et al., 'Season of birth and childhood food allergy in Australia'.

21 A. A. Ginde, et al., 'Vitamin D insufficiency in pregnant and nonpregnant women of childbearing age in the United States'.

22 C. A. Camargo, et al., 'Vitamin D status of newborns in New Zealand'.

23 N. E. Lange, et al., 'Vitamin D, the immune system and asthma'.

24 A. A. Litonjua and S. T. Weiss, 'Is vitamin D deficiency to blame for the asthma epidemic?'; S. T. Weiss, 'Bacterial components plus vitamin D: The ultimate solution to the asthma (autoimmune disease) epidemic?'.

25 M. Wjst, 'The vitamin D slant on allergy'.

26 G. Devereux, et al., 'Maternal vitamin D intake during pregnancy and early childhood wheezing'.

27 Y. Miyake, et al., 'Dairy food, calcium, and vitamin D intake in pregnancy and wheeze and eczema in infants'; M. Erkkola, et al., 'Maternal vitamin D intake during pregnancy is inversely associated with asthma and allergic rhinitis in 5-year-old children'.

28 C. R. Gale, et al., 'Maternal vitamin D status during pregnancy and child outcomes'; O. Back, et al., 'Does vitamin D intake during infancy promote the development of atopic allergy?'; E. Hypponen,

et al., 'Infant vitamin D supplementation and allergic conditions in adulthood: northern Finland birth cohort 1966'.

29 S. O. Shaheen, 'Prenatal nutrition and asthma: hope or hype?'

30 C. E. West, D. Videky and S. L. Prescott, 'Role of diet in the development of immune tolerance in the context of allergic disease'.

31 same as above.

32 M. Calvani, et al., 'Consumption of fish, butter and margarine during pregnancy and development of allergic sensitizations in the offspring: role of maternal atopy'; S. Sausenthaler, et al., 'Maternal diet during pregnancy in relation to eczema and allergic sensitization in the offspring at 2 y of age'; M. T. Salam, et al., 'Maternal fish consumption during pregnancy and risk of early childhood asthma'.

33 J. Peat, C. Salome and A. Woolcock, 'Factors associated with bronchial hyper-responsiveness in Australian adults and children'; L. Hodge, et al., 'Consumption of oily fish and childhood asthma risk'.

34 P. C. Calder, 'Dietary fatty acids and the immune system'; 'N-3 polyunsaturated fatty acids and inflammation: from molecular biology to the clinic'; and 'Polyunsaturated fatty acids, inflammation, and immunity'.

35 G. B. Marks, et al., 'Prevention of asthma during the first 5 years of life: a randomized controlled trial'.

36 N. D'Vaz, et al., 'Early postnatal fish oil supplementation in high risk infants to prevent allergy: A randomized controlled trial'.

37 J. Dunstan, et al., 'Fish oil supplementation in pregnancy modifies neonatal allergen-specific immune responses and clinical outcomes in infants at high risk of atopy: a randomised controlled trial'.

38 same as above.

39 J. A. Dunstan, et al., 'Maternal fish oil supplementation in pregnancy reduces interleukin-13 levels in cord blood of infants at high risk of atopy'.

40 J. A. Dunstan, et al., 'Fish oil supplementation in pregnancy'.

41 A. Barden, et al., 'Fish oil supplementation in pregnancy lowers F2 Isoprostanes in neonatal at high risk of atopy'.

42 J. Dunstan, et al., 'Fish oil supplementation in pregnancy'.

43 C. Furuhjelm, et al., 'Fish oil supplementation in pregnancy and lactation may decrease the risk of infant allergy'; S. F. Olsen, et al., 'Fish oil intake compared with olive oil intake in late pregnancy and asthma in the offspring: 16 y of registry-based follow-up from a randomized controlled trial'.

44 D. Palmer D, et al., 'Effect of n-3 docosahexaenoic acid (DHA) supplementation in pregnancy on infant allergies in the first year of life: a randomised controlled trial'.

45 S. L. Prescott, et al., 'Protein kinase-C zeta: a novel "protective" neonatal T cell marker that can be up-regulated by allergy prevention strategies'.

46 K. Allan, F. J. Kelly and G. Devereux, 'Antioxidants and allergic disease: a case of too little or too much?'

47 M. Utsugi, et al., 'c-Jun N-terminal kinase negatively regulates lipopolysaccharide-induced IL-12 production in human macrophages: role of mitogen-activated protein kinase in glutathione redox regulation of IL-12 production'.

48 P. H. Tan, et al., 'Inhibition of NF-kappa B and oxidative pathways in human dendritic cells by antioxidative vitamins generates regulatory T cells'.

49 C. Murr, et al., 'Antioxidants may increase the probability of developing allergic disease and asthma'.

50 P. A. Scholtens, et al., 'Fecal secretory immunoglobulin A is increased in healthy infants who receive a formula with short-chain galacto-oligosaccharides and long-chain fructo-oligosaccharides'.

51 B. Schouten, et al., 'Cow milk allergy symptoms are reduced in mice fed dietary synbiotics during oral sensitization with whey'; E. van Hoffen, et al., 'A specific mixture of short-chain galacto-oligosaccharides and long-chain fructo-oligosaccharides induces a beneficial immunoglobulin profile in infants at high risk for allergy'.

52 K. M. Maslowski, et al., 'Regulation of inflammatory responses by gut microbiota and chemoattractant receptor GPR43'.

53 S. Arslanoglu, et al., 'Early dietary intervention with a mixture of prebiotic oligosaccharides reduces the incidence of allergic manifestations and infections during the first two years of life'.

54 R. L. Miller and S. M. Ho, 'Environmental epigenetics and asthma: current concepts and call for studies'.

55 J. W. Hollingsworth, et al., 'In utero supplementation with methyl donors enhances allergic airway disease in mice'.

56 M. J. Whitrow, et al., 'Effect of supplemental folic acid in pregnancy on childhood asthma: a prospective birth cohort study'; S. E. Håberg, et al., 'Folic acid supplements in pregnancy and early childhood respiratory health'.

57 F. D. Gilliland, et al., 'Maternal smoking during pregnancy, environmental tobacco smoke exposure and childhood lung function'; M. N. Hylkema and M. J. Blacquiere, 'Intrauterine effects of maternal smoking on sensitization, asthma, and chronic obstructive pulmonary disease'.

58 P. S. Noakes, et. al., 'Maternal smoking is associated with impaired neonatal toll-like-receptor-mediated immune responses'; P. S. Noakes,

P. G. Holt and S. L. Prescott, 'Maternal smoking in pregnancy alters neonatal cytokine responses'.

59 I. M. Adcock, et al., 'Epigenetic regulation of airway inflammation'.

60 F. Perera, et al., 'Relation of DNA methylation of 5'-CpG island of ACSL3 to transplacental exposure to airborne polycyclic aromatic hydrocarbons and childhood asthma'.

61 I. Hertz-Picciotto, et al., 'Prenatal exposures to persistent and non-persistent organic compounds and effects on immune system development'.

62 P. S. Noakes, et al., 'The relationship between persistent organic pollutants in maternal and neonatal tissues and immune responses to allergens: A novel exploratory study'.

63 A. Baccarelli and V. Bollati, 'Epigenetics and environmental chemicals'.

64 K. Y. Kim, et al., 'Association of low-dose exposure to persistent organic pollutants with global DNA hypomethylation in healthy koreans'.

65 V. Daniel, et al., 'Impaired in-vitro lymphocyte responses in patients with elevated pentachlorophenol (PCP) blood levels'.

66 V. Daniel, et al., 'Associations of blood levels of PCB, HCHS, and HCB with numbers of lymphocyte subpopulations, in vitro lymphocyte response, plasma cytokine levels, and immunoglobulin autoantibodies'.

67 I. Hertz-Picciotto, et al., 'Prenatal exposures to persistent and non-persistent organic compounds and effects on immune system development'.

68 E. Reichrtova, et. al., 'Cord serum immunoglobulin E related to the environmental contamination of human placentas with organochlorine compounds'.

69 P. S. Noakes, et al.,'The relationship between persistent organic pollutants in maternal and neonatal tissues and immune responses to allergens: A novel exploratory study'.

70 I. Hertz-Picciotto, et al., 'Prenatal exposures'.

71 S. L. Prescott and K. A. Allen, 'Food Allergy: Riding the second wave of the allergy epidemic'.

72 A. A. Litonjua, et al., 'Parental history and the risk for childhood asthma. Does mother confer more risk than father?'

73 S. L. Prescott, et al., 'Effects of maternal allergen-specific IgG in cordblood on early postnatal development of allergen-specific T-cell immunity'.

74 L. A. Breckler, et al., 'Modulation of in vivo and in vitro cytokine production over the course of pregnancy in allergic and non-allergic mothers'.

75   S. L. Prescott, et al., 'Allergic women show reduced T helper type
     1 alloresponses to fetal human leucocyte antigen mismatch during
     pregnancy'.
76   B. Schaub, et al., 'Impairment of T-regulatory cells in cord blood of
     atopic mothers'; P. Amoudruz, et al., 'Neonatal immune responses to
     microbial stimuli: is there an influence of maternal allergy?'
77   M. K. Knackstedt, E. Hamelmann and P. C. Arck, 'Mothers in stress:
     consequences for the offspring'.
78   same as above.
79   S. Thavagnanam, et al., 'A meta-analysis of the association between
     Caesarean section and childhood asthma'; P. Bager, J. Wohlfahrt and
     T. Westergaard, 'Caesarean delivery and risk of atopy and allergic
     disease: meta-analyses'; M. C. Tollanes, et al., 'Cesarean section and
     risk of severe childhood asthma: a population-based cohort study';
     J. Metsala, et al., 'Perinatal factors and the risk of asthma in childhood
     – a population-based register study in Finland'.
80   M. C. Tollanes, et al., 'Cesarean section and risk of severe childhood
     asthma'.
81   T. H. Joffe and N. A. Simpson, 'Cesarean section and risk of asthma.
     The role of intrapartum antibiotics: a missing piece?'
82   T. M. McKeever, et al., 'Early exposure to infections and antibiotics
     and the incidence of allergic disease: a birth cohort study with the
     West Midlands General Practice Research Database'.
83   S. O. Shaheen, et al., 'Paracetamol use in pregnancy and wheezing
     in early childhood'; C. M. Rebordosa, et al., 'Pre-natal exposure to
     paracetamol and risk of wheezing and asthma in children: a birth
     cohort study'; H. Bisgaard, et al., 'Prenatal determinants of neonatal
     lung function in high-risk newborns'; L. Garcia-Marcos, et al., 'Is
     the effect of prenatal paracetamol exposure on wheezing in preschool
     children modified by asthma in the mother?'; V. Persky, et al.,
     'Prenatal exposure to acetaminophen and respiratory symptoms in the
     first year of life'.
84   M. Rebordosa, et al., 'Pre-natal exposure to paracetamol and risk of
     wheezing'.
85   V. Persky, et al., 'Prenatal exposure to acetaminophen'.

Chapter 9 — The practicalities: current allergy prevention strategies

1   S. L. Prescott and M. L. Tang, 'The Australasian Society of Clinical
    Immunology and Allergy position statement: summary of allergy
    prevention in children'; S. L. Prescott, M. Tang and B. Björkstén,
    'Primary allergy prevention in children 2007: a revised summary of

the Australasian Society of Clinical Immunology and Allergy Position Statement'.

2   C. Agostini. et al., 'Complementary feeding: a commentary by the ESPGHAN Committee on Nutrition'; F. R. Greer, S. H. Sicherer and A. W. Burks, 'Effects of early nutritional interventions on the development of atopic disease in infants and children: the role of maternal dietary restriction, breastfeeding, timing of introduction of complementary foods, and hydrolyzed formulas'; S. L. Prescott, et al., 'The importance of early complementary feeding in the development of oral tolerance: concerns and controversies'; A. Host, et al., 'Dietary prevention of allergic diseases in infants and small children'.

3   Infant Feeding Advice, Australasian Society of Allergy and Immunology.

4   S. L. Prescott, et al., 'The importance of early complementary feeding'.

5   N. I. Kjellman, 'Prediction and prevention of atopic allergy'; R. Zeiger et al., 'Genetic and environmental factors affecting the development of atopy through age 4 in children with atopic parents: a prospective radomised study of food allergen avoidance'.

6   A. T. Fox, et al., 'Household peanut consumption as a risk factor for the development of peanut allergy'.

7   M. S. Kramer, 'Maternal antigen avoidance during pregnancy for preventing atopic disease in infants of women at high risk'; K. Fälth-Magnusson and N-I. Kjellman, 'Allergy prevention by maternal elimination diet during late pregnancy - a five year follow-up of a randomised trial'.

8   A. Woodcock, et al., 'Early life environmental control: effect on symptoms, sensitization, and lung function at age 3 years'; G. B. Marks, et al., 'Prevention of asthma during the first 5 years of life: a randomized controlled trial'.

9   B. Hesselmar, et al., 'Does early exposure to cat or dog protect against later allergy development?'; D. R. Ownby, C. C. Johnson, E. L. Peterson, 'Exposure to dogs and cats in the first year of life and risk of allergic sensitization at 6 to 7 years of age'; G. Anyo et al., 'Early, current and past pet ownership: associations with sensitization, bronchial responsiveness and allergic symptoms in school children'.

10 T. A. Platts-Mills, et al., 'Relevance of early or current pet ownership to the prevalence of allergic diseases'.

11 G. Lilja, et al., 'Effects of maternal diet during late pregnancy and lactation on the development of atopic diseases in infants up to 18 months of age – in-vivo results'; N. Sigurs, G. Hattevig and B. Kjellman, 'Maternal avoidance of eggs, cow's milk, and fish during lactation: effect on allergic manifestations, skin-prick tests, and specific

IgE antibodies in children at age 4 years'; G. Hattevig, N. Sigurs and B. Kjellman, 'Effects of maternal dietary avoidance during lactation on allergy in children at 10 years of age'.

12 D. M. Fergusson, L. J. Horwood and F. T. Shannon, 'Risk factors in childhood eczema'; J. S. Forsyth et al., 'Relation between early introduction of solid food to infants and their weight and illnesses during the first two years of life'; M. Kajosaari and U. M. Saarinen, 'Prophylaxis of atopic disease by six months' total solid food elimination. Evaluation of 135 exclusively breast-fed infants of atopic families'; J. Morgan, et al., 'Eczema and early solid feeding in preterm infants'; A. C. Wilson, et al., 'Relation of infant diet to childhood health: seven year follow up of cohort of children in Dundee infant feeding study'; A. Zutavern, et al., 'Timing of solid food introduction in relation to atopic dermatitis and atopic sensitization: results from a prospective birth cohort study'.

13 B. Filipiak, et al., 'Solid food introduction in relation to eczema: results from a four-year prospective birth cohort study'.

14 J. A. Poole, et al., 'Timing of initial exposure to cereal grains and the risk of wheat allergy'; A. Zutavern, et al., 'The introduction of solids in relation to asthma and eczema'; B. Filipiak, et al. 'Solid food introduction in relation to eczema'.

15 J. M. Norris, et al., 'Risk of celiac disease autoimmunity and timing of gluten introduction in the diet of infants at increased risk of disease'.

16 C. Agostoni, et al., 'Complementary feeding'; F. R. Greer, S. H. Sicherer and A. W. Burks, 'Effects of early nutritional interventions'; S. L. Prescott, et al., 'The importance of early complementary feeding'; A. Host, et al., 'Dietary prevention of allergic diseases'.

17 American Academy of Pediatrics, Committee on Nutrition, 'Hypoallergenic infant formulas'.

18 Department of Nutrition for Health and Development WHO, 'The optimal duration of exclusive breastfeeding: report of an expert consultation'.

19 C. Agostoni, et al., 'Complementary feeding'; F. R. Greer, et al., 'Effects of early nutritional interventions'; S. L. Prescott, et al., 'The importance of early complementary feeding'; A. Host, et al., 'Dietary prevention of allergic diseases'.

20 American Academy of Pediatrics, Committee on Nutrition, 'Hypoallergenic infant formulas'.

21 Infant Feeding Advice, Australasian Society of Allergy and Immunology.

22 A. von Berg, et al., 'Preventive effect of hydrolyzed infant formulas persists until age 6 years: Long-term results from the German Infant

Nutritional Intervention Study (GINI)'; D. Osborn and J.Sinn, 'Formulas containing hydrolysed protein for prevention of allergy and food intolerance in infants'.

23 A. von Berg, et al., 'Preventive effect of hydrolyzed infant formulas'; D. Osborn and J. Sinn, 'Formulas containing hydrolysed protein'.

24 Infant Feeding Advice, Australasian Society of Allergy and Immunology.

25 S. Halken, et al., 'Passive smoking as a risk factor for development of obstructive respiratory disease and allergic sensitization'; F. Martinez, A. Wright, L. Taussig, et al., 'Asthma and wheezing in the first six years of life'.

26 M. Kalliomäki, et al., 'Probiotics in primary prevention of atopic disease: a randomised placebo-controlled trial'.

27 M. Kalliomäki, et al., 'Probiotics and prevention of atopic disease: 4-year follow-up of a randomised placebo-controlled trial'; M. Kalliomäki, et al., 'Probiotics during the first 7 years of life: a cumulative risk reduction of eczema in a randomized, placebo-controlled trial'.

28 These studies are summarised in H. Johannsen and S. L. Prescott, 'Practical prebiotics, probiotics and synbiotics for allergists: how useful are they?'

29 M. V. Kopp, et al., 'Randomized, double-blind, placebo-controlled trial of probiotics for primary prevention: no clinical effects of *Lactobacillus* GG supplementation'.

30 A. L. Taylor, J. A. Dunstan and S. L. Prescott, 'Probiotic supplementation for the first 6 months of life fails to reduce the risk of atopic dermatitis and increases the risk of allergen sensitization in high-risk children: a randomized controlled trial'.

31 same as above.

32 D. Osborn and J. Sinn, 'Probiotics in infants for prevention of allergic disease and food hypersensitivity'.

33 As reviewed in C. E. West, D. Videky and S. L. Prescott, 'Role of diet zin the development of immune tolerance in the context of allergic disease'.

34 S. Arslanoglu, et al., 'Early dietary intervention with a mixture of prebiotic oligosaccharides reduces the incidence of allergic manifestations and infections during the first two years of life'; G. Moro, et al., 'A mixture of prebiotic oligosaccharides reduces the incidence of atopic dermatitis during the first six months of age'.

35 G. Moro, et al., 'A mixture of prebiotic oligosaccharides'.

36 S. Arslanoglu, et al., 'Early dietary intervention'.

37 As reviewed in C. E. West, D. Videky and S. L. Prescott, 'Role of diet

in the development of immune tolerance'.

38 J. Dunstan, et al., 'Fish oil supplementation in pregnancy modifies
    neonatal allergen-specific immune responses and clinical outcomes in
    infants at high risk of atopy: a randomised controlled trial'; S. F. Olsen,
    et al., 'Fish oil intake compared with olive oil intake in late pregnancy
    and asthma in the offspring: 16 y of registry-based follow-up
    from a randomized controlled trial'; C. Furuhjelm, et al., 'Fish oil
    supplementation in pregnancy and lactation may decrease the risk of
    infant allergy'.

39 D. Palmer, et al., 'Effect of n-3 docosahexaenoic acid (DHA)
    supplementation in pregnancy on infant allergies in the first year of
    life: a randomised controlled trial'.

40 G. McGwin, J. Lienert and J. I. Kennedy, 'Formaldehyde exposure
    and asthma in children: a systematic review'; P. Wolkoff and G. D.
    Nielsen, 'Non-cancer effects of formaldehyde and relevance for setting
    an indoor air guideline'.

41 A. L. Ponsonby, et al., 'A prospective study of the association between
    home gas appliance use during infancy and subsequent dust mite
    sensitization and lung function in childhood'.

42 M. B. Aldous, et al., 'Evaporative cooling and other home factors and
    lower respiratory tract illness during the first year of life'.

43 S. L. Prescott and M. L. Tang, 'The Australasian Society of Clinical
    Immunology and Allergy position statement'.

44 G. B. Pajno, et al., 'Prevention of new sensitisations in asthmatic
    children monosensitised to house dust mite by specific
    immunotherapy. A six year follow-up study'.

Chapter 10 — Allergy in practice: general principles of diagnosis and management

1 A. J. Frew, 'Hundred years of allergen immunotherapy'.
2 H. S. Ami, G. M. Liss and D. I. Bernstein, 'Evaluation of near-fatal
   reactions to allergen immunotherapy injections'.
3 same as above
4 J. M. Weiner, 'Allergen injection immunotherapy'.
5 C. Möller, et al., 'Pollen immunotherapy reduces the development of
   asthma in children with seasonal rhinoconjunctivitis (the PAT-study)'.
6 G. B. Pajno, et al., 'Prevention of new sensitisations in asthmatic
   children monosensitised to house dust mite by specific
   immunotherapy. A six year follow-up study'.

Chapter 11 — Food allergy – the new allergy epidemic

1 World Allergy Organization (WAO), White Book on Allergy.

2   same as above.

3   R. J. Mullins, 'Paediatric food allergy trends in a community-based specialist allergy practice, 1995–2006'.

4   H. A. Sampson, 'Food allergy'.

5   N. J. Osborne, et al., 'Prevalence of challenge-proven IgE-mediated food allergy using population-based sampling and predetermined challenge criteria in infants'.

6   R. J. Mullins, 'Paediatric food allergy trends'.

7   J. Grundy, et al., 'Rising prevalence of allergy to peanut in children: Data from 2 sequential cohorts'.

8   K. J. Allen, D. J. Hill and R. G. Heine, 'Food allergy in childhood'.

9   J. M. Skripak, et al., 'The natural history of IgE-mediated cow's milk allergy'; J. H. Savage, et al., 'The natural history of egg allergy'.

10 A. T. Schofield, 'A case of egg poisoning'.

11 M. Calvani, V. Giorgio and S. Miceli Sopo, 'Specific oral tolerance induction for food. A systematic review'.

12 A. Nowak-Wegrzyn, et al., 'Food protein induced enterocolitis syndrome caused by solid food proteins'.

13 K. A. Allen, et al., 'Management of cow's milk protein allergy in infants and young children: An expert panel perspective'.

14 A. Fiocchi, et al., 'World Allergy Organization (WAO) diagnosis and rationale for action against cow's milk allergy (DRACMA) guidelines'.

15 same as above.

16 K. A. Allen, et al., 'Management of cow's milk protein allergy in infants and young children'.

17 same as above.

18 same as above.

19 same as above.

20 same as above.

Chapter 12 — Eczema and atopic dermatitis

1   R. J. Mullins, 'Paediatric food allergy trends in a community-based specialist allergy practice, 1995–2006'.

2   M. I. Asher, et al., 'Worldwide time trends in the prevalence of symptoms of asthma, allergic rhinoconjunctivitis, and eczema in childhood: ISAAC Phases One and Three repeat multicountry cross-sectional surveys'.

3   S. Brown and N. J. Reynolds, 'Atopic and non-atopic eczema (Clinical Review)'.

4   D. Y. M. Leung, et al., 'New insights into atopic dermatitis'.

5   M. J. Cork, et al., 'Epidermal barrier dysfunction in atopic dermatitis'.

6   S. Brown and N. J. Reynolds, 'Atopic and non-atopic eczema'.
7   C. H. Katelaris and J. E. Peake, 'Allergy and the skin: eczema and chronic urticaria'.
8   same as above.
9   D. J. Atherton, 'Topical corticosteroids in atopic dermatitis'.
10 J. T. Huang, et al., 'Treatment of Staphylococcus aureus colonization in atopic dermatitis decreases disease severity'.
11 K. J. Allen, D. J. Hill and R. G. Heine, 'Food allergy in childhood'.

Chapter 13 — Asthma

1   World Health Organisation, 'Global surveillance, prevention and control of chronic respiratory diseases: a comprehensive approach'.
2   World Allergy Organization, 'White Book on Allergy'.
3   C. Robertson, et al., 'Asthma and other atopic diseases in Australian children'; M. I. Asher, et al., 'Worldwide time trends in the prevalence of symptoms of asthma, allergic rhinoconjunctivitis, and eczema in childhood: ISAAC Phases One and Three repeat multicountry cross-sectional surveys'.
4   C. F. Robertson, M.F. Roberts, and J.H. Kappers, 'Asthma prevalence in Melbourne schoolchildren: have we reached the peak?'
5   M. I. Asher et al., 'Worldwide time trends in the prevalence of symptoms'.
6   'Asthma management handbook', National Asthma Council Australia Ltd.
7   same as above.
8   same as above.
9   same as above.
10 same as above.
11 J. H. Wildhaber, et al., 'Aerosol delivery to wheezy infants: a comparison between a nebulizer and two small volume spacers'.
12 'Asthma management handbook.' National Asthma Council Australia Ltd.

Chapter 14 — Allergic rhinitis and allergic rhinoconjunctivitis

1   'The economic impact of allergic disease in Australia: not to be sneezed at.' Report by Access Economics Pty Ltd for the Australasian Society of Clinical Immunology and Allergy (ASCIA), 2007.
2   J. Bostock, 'Case of a periodical affection of the eyes and chest'.
3   J. Bostock, 'On the cattarhus aestivus or summer catarrh'.
4   J. L. Hopper et al., 'Increase in the self-reported prevalence of asthma and hay fever in adults over the last generation: a matched parent-offspring study'.

5   C. Robertson et al., 'Asthma and other atopic diseases in Australian children (Australian arm of the International Study of Asthma and Allergy in Childhood)'.

6   C. F. Robertson, M.F. Roberts, J.H. Kappers, 'Asthma prevalence in Melbourne schoolchildren: have we reached the peak?'

7   N. Ait-Khaled et al., 'Global map of the prevalence of symptoms of rhinoconjunctivitis in children: The International Study of Asthma and Allergies in Childhood (ISAAC) Phase Three'; M. I. Asher et al., 'Worldwide time trends in the prevalence of symptoms of asthma, allergic rhinoconjunctivitis, and eczema in childhood: ISAAC Phases One and Three repeat multicountry cross-sectional surveys'.

8   J. A. Denburg and S. F. van Eeden, 'Bone marrow progenitors in inflammation and repair: new vistas in respiratory biology and pathophysiology'.

9   S. Hazarika, R. M. van Scott and R. M. Lust, 'Myocardial ischemia-reperfusion injury is enhanced in a model of systemic allergy and asthma'; S. Onufrak, J. Abramson and V. Vaccarino, 'Adult-onset asthma is associated with increased carotid atherosclerosis among women in the atherosclerosis risk in communities (ARIC) study'.

10   S. Suissa et al., 'Inhaled corticosteroid use in asthma and the prevention of myocardial infarction'.

11   J. Bousquet, P. van Cauwenberge and N. Khaltaev, 'Allergic rhinitis and its impact on asthma'.

12   same as above.

13   R. S. Walls et al., 'Optimising the management of allergic rhinitis: an Australian perspective'.

14   same as above.

15   same as above.

16   C. Moller et al., 'Safety of nasal budesonide in the long-term treatment of children with perennial rhinitis'.

17   R. S. Walls et al., 'Optimising the management of allergic rhinitis: an Australian perspective'.

Chapter 15 — Other assorted allergies

1   F. C. K. Thien, 'Drug hypersensitivity'.

2   C. H. Katelaris and J. E. Peake, 'Allergy and the skin: eczema and chronic urticaria'.

3   M. W. Greaves, 'The skin as target for IgE-mediated allergic reactions: Chronic urticaria in childhood'.

4   same as above.

BIBLIOGRAPHY

Aberg, N., B. Hesselmar, B. Aberg, B. Eriksson, 'Increase of asthma, allergic rhinitis and eczema in Swedish schoolchildren between 1979 and 1991', *Clinical & Experimental Allergy*, 1995, vol. 25, pp. 815–19.

Adcock, I. M., L. Tsaprouni, P. Bhavsar, K. Ito, 'Epigenetic regulation of airway inflammation', *Current Opinion in Immunology*, 2007, no. 19, pp. 694–700.

Agostoni, C., T. Decsi, M. Fewtrell, O. Goulet, S. Kolacek, B. Koletzko, et al., 'Complementary feeding: a commentary by the ESPGHAN Committee on Nutrition', *Journal of Pediatric Gastroenterology and Nutrition*, 2008, no. 46, pp. 99–110.

Ait-Khaled, N., N. Pearce, H. R. Anderson, P. Ellwood, S. Montefort, J. Shah, 'Global map of the prevalence of symptoms of rhinoconjunctivitis in children: The International Study of Asthma and Allergies in Childhood (ISAAC) Phase Three', *Allergy*, 2009, no. 64, pp. 123–48.

Aldous, M. B., C. J. Holberg, A. L. Wright, F. D. Martinez, L. M. Taussig, 'Evaporative cooling and other home factors and lower respiratory tract illness during the first year of life', Group Health Medical Associates, *American Journal of Epidemiology*, 1996, no. 143, pp. 423–30.

Allen, K. A., G. P. Davidson, A. S. Day, D. J. Hill, A. S. Kemp, J. E. Peake, et al., 'Management of cow's milk protein allergy in infants and young children: An expert panel perspective', *Journal of Paediatrics and Child Health*, 2009, no. 45, pp. 481–6.

Allen, K. J., D. J. Hill, R. G. Heine, 'Food allergy in childhood', *The Medical Journal of Australia*, 2006, no. 185, pp. 394–400.

Allan, K., F. J. Kelly, G. Devereux, 'Antioxidants and allergic disease: a case of too little or too much?', *Clinical & Experimental Allergy*, 2010, no. 40, pp. 370–80.

Aluvihare, V. R., M. Kallikourdis, A. G. Betz, 'Regulatory T cells mediate maternal tolerance to the fetus', *National Immunology*, 2004, vol. 5, no. 3, pp. 266–71.

American Academy of Pediatrics, Committee on Nutrition, 'Hypoallergenic infant formulas', *Pediatrics*, 2000, vol. 106, pp. 346–9.

Amin, H. S., G. M. Liss, D. I. Bernstein, 'Evaluation of near-fatal reactions to allergen immunotherapy injections', *Journal of Allergy and Clinical Immunology*, 2006, vol. 117, pp. 169–75.

Amoudruz, P., U. Holmlund, S. Saghafian-Hedengren, C. Nilsson, E. Sverremark-Ekström, 'Impaired Toll-like receptor 2 signalling in monocytes from 5-year-old allergic children', *Clinical & Experimental Immunology*, 2009, no. 155, pp. 387–94.

Amoudruz, P., U. Holmlund, V. Malmstrom, C. Trollmo, K. Bremme, A. Scheynius, et al., 'Neonatal immune responses to microbial stimuli: is there an influence of maternal allergy?', *Journal of Allergy and Clinical Immunology*, 2005, no. 115, pp. 1304–10.

Anyo, G., B. Brunekreef, G. de Meer, F. Aarts, N. A. Janssen, P. van Vliet P, 'Early, current and past pet ownership: associations with sensitization, bronchial responsiveness and allergic symptoms in school children', *Clinical & Experimental Immunology*, 2002, no. 32, pp. 361–6.

Armitage, E., H. E. Drummond, D. C. Wilson, S. Ghosh, 'Increasing incidence of both juvenile-onset Crohn's disease and ulcerative colitis in Scotland, *European Journal of Gastroenterology & Hepatology*, 2001, vol. 13, pp. 1439–47.

Arslanoglu, S., G. E. Moro, J. Schmitt, L. Tandoi, S. Rizzardi, G. Boehm, 'Early dietary intervention with a mixture of prebiotic oligosaccharides reduces the incidence of allergic manifestations and infections during the first two years of life', *Journal of Nutrition*, 2008, vol. 138, no. 6, pp. 1091–5.

Asher, M. I., S. Montefort, B. Bjorksten, C. K. Lai, D. P. Strachan, S. K.

Weiland, et al., 'Worldwide time trends in the prevalence of symptoms of asthma, allergic rhinoconjunctivitis, and eczema in childhood: ISAAC Phases One and Three repeat multicountry cross-sectional surveys', *Lancet*, 2006, no. 368, pp. 733–43.

Asthma Management Handbook, National Asthma Council Australia Ltd., Melbourne, Australia, 2006.

Atherton, D. J., 'Topical corticosteroids in atopic dermatitis', *BMJ*, 2003, no. 327, pp. 942–3.

Baccarelli, A., V. Bollati, 'Epigenetics and environmental chemicals', *Current Opinion in Pediatrics*, 2009, no. 21, pp. 243–51.

Bach, J. F., 'The effect of infections on susceptibility to autoimmune and allergic diseases', *The New England Journal of Medicine*, 2002, no. 347, pp. 911–20.

Back, O., H. K. Blomquist, O. Hernell, B. Stenberg, 'Does vitamin D intake during infancy promote the development of atopic allergy?', *Acta Dermito-venereologica*, 2009, no. 89, pp. 28–32.

Bager, P., J. Wohlfahrt, T. Westergaard, 'Caesarean delivery and risk of atopy and allergic disease: meta-analyses', *Clinical & Experimental Allergy*, 2008, no. 38, pp. 634–42.

Baldini, M., I. C. Lohman, M. Halonen, R. P. Erickson, P. G. Holt, F. D. Martinez, 'A Polymorphism in the 5' flanking region of the CD14 gene is associated with circulating soluble CD14 levels and with total serum immunoglobulin E', *American Journal of Respiratory Cell and Molecular Biology*, 1999, no. 20, pp.976–83.

Barden, A., T. A. Mori, J. A. Dunstan, A. L. Taylor, C. A. Thornton, K. D. Croft, et al., 'Fish oil supplementation in pregnancy lowers F2 Isoprostanes in neonatal at high risk of atopy', *Free Radical Research*, 2004, vol. 38, no. 3, pp. 233–9.

Barker, D. J., 'Fetal origins of coronary heart disease', *British Medical Journal*, 1995, no. 311, pp. 171–4.

Barker, D., P. Winter, C. Osmond, B. Margetts, S. Simmonds, 'Weight in infancy and death from ischemic heart disease', *Lancet*, 1989, no. ii, p. 577.

Bennett C. L., J. Christie, F. Ramsdell, M. E. Brunkow, P. J. Ferguson, L. Whitesell, et al., 'The immune dysregulation, polyendocrinopathy, enteropathy, X-linked syndrome (IPEX) is caused by mutations of FOXP3', *Nature Genetics*, 2001, no. 27, pp. 20–1.

Bisgaard, H., L. Loland, K. K. Holst, C. B. Pipper, 'Prenatal determinants of neonatal lung function in high-risk newborns', *Journal of Allergy and Clinical Immunology*, 2009.

Björkstén, B., 'The gut microbiota: a complex ecosystem', *Clinical & Experimental Allergy*, 2006, no. 36, pp. 1215-17.

Björkstén, B., E. Sepp, K. Julge, T. Voor, M. Mikelsaar, 'Allergy development and the intestinal microflora during the first year of life', *Journal of Allergy and Clinical Immunology*, 2001, no. 108, pp. 516–20.

Blumer, N., S. Sel, S. Virna, C. C. Patrascan, S. Zimmermann, U. Herz et al., 'Perinatal maternal application of *Lactobacillus rhamnosus* GG suppresses allergic airway inflammation in mouse offspring', *Clinical & Experimental Allergy*, 2007, no. 37, pp. 348–57.

Blumer, N., U. Herz, M. Wegmann, H. Renz, 'Prenatal lipopolysaccharide-exposure prevents allergic sensitisation and airway inflammation, but not airway responsiveness in a murine model of experimental asthma', *Clinical & Experimental Allergy*, 2005, no. 35, pp. 397–402.

Bostock, J., 'Case of a periodical affection of the eyes and chest', *Medico-Chirurgical Transactions*, 1819, no. 10, pp. 161–2.

—— 'On the cattarhus aestivus or summer catarrh', *Medico-Chirurgical Transactions*, 1828, no. 14, pp. 437–46.

Bottcher, M. F., E. K. Nordin, A. Sandin, T. Midtvedt, B. Bjorksten, 'Microflora-associated characteristics in faeces from allergic and nonallergic infants', *Clinical & Experimental Allergy*, 2000, no. 30, pp. 1591–6.

Bousquet, J., P. van Cauwenberge, N. Khaltaev, 'Allergic rhinitis and its impact on asthma', *Journal of Allergy and Clinical Immunology*, 2001, no. 108, pp. S147–334.

Breckler, L. A., J. Hale, W. Jung, L. Westcott, J. A. Dunstan, C. A. Thornton, et al., 'Modulation of in vivo and in vitro cytokine production over the course of pregnancy in allergic and non-allergic mothers', *Pediatric Allergy and Immunology*, 2010, no. 21, pp. 14–21.

Brown, S., N. J. Reynolds, 'Atopic and non-atopic eczema (Clinical Review)', *BMJ*, 2006, pp. 584–8.

Calder, P. C., 'Dietary fatty acids and the immune system', *Nutrition Reviews*, 1998, no. 56, pp. S70–83.

—— 'Polyunsaturated fatty acids, inflammation, and immunity', *Lipids*, 2001, no. 36, pp. 1007–24.

—— 'N-3 polyunsaturated fatty acids and inflammation: from molecular biology to the clinic', *Lipids*, 2003, no. 38, pp. 343–52.

Calvani, M., C. Alessandri, S. M. Sopo, V. Panetta, G. Pingitore, S. Tripodi, et al., 'Consumption of fish, butter and margarine during pregnancy and development of allergic sensitizations in the off-spring: role of maternal atopy', *Pediatric Allergy and Immunology*, 2006, no. 17, pp. 94–102.

Calvani, M., V. Giorgio, S. Miceli Sopo, 'Specific oral tolerance induction for food. A systematic review', *European Annals of Allergy and Clinical Immunology*, 2010, no. 42, pp. 11–9.

Camargo, C. A. Jr., S. Clark, M. S. Kaplan, P. Lieberman, R. A. Wood, 'Regional differences in EpiPen prescriptions in the United States: the potential role of vitamin D', *Journal of Allergy and Clinical Immunology*, 2007, no. 120, pp. 131–6.

Camargo, C. A., Jr., T. Ingham, K. Wickens, R. I. Thadhani, K. M. Silvers, M. J. Epton, et al., 'Vitamin D status of newborns in New Zealand', *British Journal of Nutrition*, 2010, no. 104, pp. 1051–7.

Carr, R. D., M. Berke, S. W. Becker, 'Incidence in atopy in the general population', *Archives of Dermatology*, 1964, vol. 89, p. 27.

Cookson, W. O. C. M., P. A. Sharp, J. A. Faux, J. M. Hopkin, 'Linkage between Immunoglobulin E responses underlying asthma and rhinitis and chromosome 11q', *Lancet*, 1989, no. 1 (8650), pp.1292–4

Cork, M. J., S. G. Danby, Y. Vasilopoulos, J. Hadgraft, M. E. Lane, M. Moustafa, et al., 'Epidermal barrier dysfunction in atopic dermatitis', *Journal of Investigative Dermatology*, 2009, no. 129, pp. 1892–908.

Danchenko, N., J. A. Satia, M. S. Anthony, 'Epidemiology of systemic lupus erythematosus: a comparison of worldwide disease burden', *Lupus*, 2006, vol. 15, pp. 308–18.

Daniel, V., W. Huber, K. Bauer, G. Opelz, 'Impaired in-vitro lymphocyte responses in patients with elevated pentachlorophenol (PCP) blood levels', *Archives of Environmental Health*, 1995, vol. 50, no.4, pp. 287–92.

Daniel, V., W. Huber, K. Bauer, C. Suesal, C. Conradt, G. Opelz, 'Associations of blood levels of PCB, HCHS, and HCB with numbers of lymphocyte subpopulations, in vitro lymphocyte response, plasma cytokine levels, and immunoglobulin autoantibodies', *Environmental Health Perspectives*, 2001, vol. 109, no. 2, pp. 173–8.

Denburg, J. A., S. F. van Eeden, 'Bone marrow progenitors in inflammation and repair: new vistas in respiratory biology and pathophysiology', *European Respiratory Journal*, 2006, no. 27, pp.441–5.

Department of Nutrition for Health and Development WHO, 'The optimal duration of exclusive breastfeeding: report of an expert consultation', WHO/NHD/ 01.09.2002 2001, available at <http://www.who.int/child-adolescent-health/New_Publications/NUTRITION/WHO_CAH_01_24.pdf>

Devereux, G., A. A. Litonjua, S. W. Turner, L. C. Craig, G. McNeill, S. Martindale, et al., 'Maternal vitamin D intake during pregnancy and early childhood wheezing', *The American Journal of Clinical Nutrition*, 2007, no. 85, pp. 853–9.

Dunstan, J., T. A. Mori, A. Barden, L. J. Beilin, A. Taylor, P. G. Holt, et al., 'Fish oil supplementation in pregnancy modifies neonatal allergen-specific immune responses and clinical outcomes in infants at high risk of atopy: a randomised controlled trial', *Journal of Allergy and Clinical Immunology*, 2003, no. 112, pp. 1178–84.

——'Maternal fish oil supplementation in pregnancy reduces interleukin-13 levels in cord blood of infants at high risk of atopy', *Clinical & Experimental Allergy*, 2003, no. 33, pp. 442–8.

D'Vaz, N., Y. Ma, J. A. Dunstan, C. Hii, S. Meldrum, A. Ferrante, et al.,

'Neonatal T cell protein kinase C zeta as a screening test for predicting allergic disease and disease severity', forthcoming.

D'Vaz, N., S. J. Meldrum, J. A. Dunstan, D. Martino, S. McCarthy, J. Metcalfe, et al., 'Early postnatal fish oil supplementation in high risk infants to prevent allergy: A randomized controlled trial', forthcoming.

Eder, W., W. Klimecki, L. Yu, E. von Mutius, J. Riedler, C. Braun-Fahrlander et al., 'Opposite effects of CD 14/-260 on serum IgE levels in children raised in different environments', *Journal of Allergy and Clinical Immunology*, 2005, no. 116, pp. 601–7.

Erkkola, M., M. Kaila, B. I. Nwaru, C. Kronberg-Kippila, S. Ahonen, J. Nevalainen, et al., 'Maternal vitamin D intake during pregnancy is inversely associated with asthma and allergic rhinitis in 5-year-old children', *Clinical & Experimental Allergy*, 2009, no. 39, pp. 875–82.

Fälth-Magnusson, K., N-I. Kjellman, 'Allergy prevention by maternal elimination diet during late pregnancy - a five year follow-up of a randomised trial', *Journal of Allergy and Clinical Immunology*, 1992, no. 89, pp. 709–13.

Fergusson, D. M., L. J. Horwood, F. T. Shannon, 'Risk factors in childhood eczema', *Journal of Epidemiology and Community Health*, 1982, no. 36, pp. 118–22.

Filipiak, B., A. Zutavern, S. Koletzko, A. von Berg, I. Brockow, A. Grubl, et al., 'Solid food introduction in relation to eczema: results from a four-year prospective birth cohort study', *Journal of Pediatrics*, 2007, no. 151, pp. 352–8.

Fiocchi, A., J. Brozek, H. Schunemann, S. L. Bahna, A. von Berg, K. Beyer, et al., 'World Allergy Organization (WAO) Diagnosis and Rationale for Action against Cow's Milk Allergy (DRACMA) Guidelines', *Paediatric Allergy and Immunology*, 2010, no. 21, Suppl. 21, pp. 1–125.

Forsyth, J. S., S. A. Ogston, A. Clark, C. D. Florey, P. W. Howie. 'Relation between early introduction of solid food to infants and their weight and illnesses during the first two years of life', *BMJ*, 1993, no. 306, pp. 1572–6.

Fox, A. T., P. Sasieni, G. du Toit, H. Syed, G. Lack, 'Household peanut consumption as a risk factor for the development of peanut allergy', *Journal of Allergy and Clinical Immunology*, 2009, no. 123, pp. 417–23.

Frew, A. J., 'Hundred years of allergen immunotherapy', *Clinical & Experimental Allergy*, 2011.

Furuhjelm, C., K. Warstedt, J. Larsson, M. Fredriksson, M. F. Bottcher, K. Falth-Magnusson, et al., 'Fish oil supplementation in pregnancy and lactation may decrease the risk of infant allergy', *Acta Paediatrica*, 2009, vol. 98, no. 9, pp. 1461–7.

Gale, C. R., S. M. Robinson, N. C. Harvey, M. K. Javaid, B. Jiang, C. N. Martyn, et al., 'Maternal vitamin D status during pregnancy and child outcomes', *European Journal of Clinical Nutrition*, 2008, no. 62, pp. 68–77.

Gale, E. A. M., 'The rise of childhood type 1 diabetes in the twentieth century, *Diabetes*, 2002, vol. 51, pp. 3353–61.

Gao, P. S., X. Q. Mao, M. Baldini, M. H. Roberts, C. N. Adra, T. Shirakawa et al., 'Serum total IgE levels and CD14 on chromosome 5q31', *Clinical Genetics*, 1999, no. 56, pp.164–5.

Garcia-Marcos, L., M. Sanchez-Solis, V. Perez-Fernandez, M. D. Pastor-Vivero, P. Mondejar-Lopez, J. Valverde-Molina, 'Is the Effect of Prenatal Paracetamol Exposure on Wheezing in Preschool Children Modified by Asthma in the Mother?', *International Archives of Allergy and Immunology*, 2008, no. 149, pp. 33–7.

Gilliland, F.D., K. Berhane, R. McConnell, W. J. Gauderman, H. Vora, E. B. Rappaport, et al., 'Maternal smoking during pregnancy, environmental tobacco smoke exposure and childhood lung function', *Thorax*, 2000, no. 55, pp. 271–6.

Ginde, A. A., A. F. Sullivan, J. M. Mansbach, C. A. Camargo Jr. 'Vitamin D insufficiency in pregnant and nonpregnant women of childbearing age in the United States,' *American Journal of Obstetrics and Gynecology*, 2010, no. 202, pp. 436 e1–8.

Greaves, M. W., 'The skin as target for IgE-mediated allergic reactions: Chronic urticaria in childhood', *Allergy*, 2000, no. 55, pp. 309–20.

Greer, F. R., S. H. Sicherer, A. W. Burks, 'Effects of early nutritional interventions on the development of atopic disease in infants and children: the role of maternal dietary restriction, breastfeeding, timing of introduction of complementary foods, and hydrolyzed formulas', *Pediatrics*, 2008, no. 121, pp. 183–91.

Grundy, J., S. Matthews, B. Bateman, T. Dean, S. H. Arshad, 'Rising prevalence of allergy to peanut in children: Data from 2 sequential cohorts', *Journal of Allergy and Clinical Immunology*, 2002, no. 110, pp. 784–9.

Håberg, S. E., S. J. London, H. Stigum, P. Nafstad, W. Nystad, 'Folic acid supplements in pregnancy and early childhood respiratory health', *Archives of Disease in Childhood*, 2009, no. 94, pp. 180–4.

Halken, S., A. Høst, L. Nilsson, E. Taudorf, 'Passive smoking as a risk factor for development of obstructive respiratory disease and allergic sensitization', *Allergy*, 1995, no. 50, pp. 97–105.

Hanson, M., P. Gluckman, 'Developmental origins of noncommunicable disease: population and public health implications', *American Journal of Clinical Nutrition*, 2011, ePub forthcoming.

Hattevig, G., N. Sigurs, B. Kjellman, E'ffects of maternal dietary avoidance during lactation on allergy in children at 10 years of age', *Acta Paediatrica*, 1999, no. 88, pp. 7–12.

Hazarika, S., M. R. van Scott, R. M. Lust, 'Myocardial ischemia-reperfusion injury is enhanced in a model of systemic allergy and asthma', *American Journal of Physiology – Heart and Circulatory Physiology*, 2004, no. 286, pp. H1720–5.

Herbert, O. C., R. S. Barnetson, W. Weninger, U. Kramer, H. Behrendt, J. Ring, 'Western lifestyle and increased prevalence of atopic diseases: An example from a small Papua New Guinean island', *World Allergy Organization Journal*, 2009, pp. 130–7.

Hertz-Picciotto, I., H. Y. Park, M. Dostal, A. Kocan, T. Trnovec, R. Sram, 'Prenatal exposures to persistent and non-persistent organic compounds and effects on immune system development', *Basic & Clinical Pharmacology and Toxicology*, 2008, no. 102, pp. 146–54.

Hesselmar, B., N. Åberg, B. Åberg, B. Eriksson, B. Björkstén, 'Does early exposure to cat or dog protect against later allergy development?', *Clinical & Experimental Allergy*, 1999, no. 29, pp. 611–7.

Hodge, L., C. Salome, J. Peat, M. Haby, W. Xuan, A. Woolcock, 'Consumption of oily fish and childhood asthma risk', *The Medical Journal of Australia*, 1996, no. 164, pp. 137–40.

Hollingsworth, J. W., S. Maruoka, K. Boon, S. Garantziotis, Z. Li, J. Tomfohr, et al., 'In utero supplementation with methyl donors enhances allergic airway disease in mice', *Journal of Clinical Investigation*, 2008, no. 118, pp. 3462–9.

Holt, P. G., P. D. Sly, 'Interactions between respiratory tract infections and atopy in the aetiology of asthma', *European Respiratory Journal*, 2002, no. 19, pp. 538–45.

Hopper, J. L., M. A. Jenkins, J. B. Carlin, G. G. Giles, 'Increase in the self-reported prevalence of asthma and hay fever in adults over the last generation: a matched parent-offspring study', *Australian Journal of Public Health*, 1995, no. 19, pp. 120–4.

Host, A., S. Halken, A. Muraro, S. Dreborg, B. Niggemann, R. Aalberse, et al., 'Dietary prevention of allergic diseases in infants and small children', *Pediatric Allergy and Immunology*, 2008, no. 19, pp. 1–4.

Huang, J. T., M. Abrams, B. Tlougan, A. Rademaker, A. S. Paller, 'Treatment of Staphylococcus aureus colonization in atopic dermatitis decreases disease severity', *Pediatrics*, 2009, no. 123, pp. e808–14.

Hylkema, M. N., M. J. Blacquiere, 'Intrauterine effects of maternal smoking on sensitization, asthma, and chronic obstructive pulmonary disease', *Proceedings of the American Thoracic Society*, 2009, no. 6, pp. 660–2.

Hypponen, E., U. Sovio, M. Wjst, S. Patel, J. Pekkanen, A. L. Hartikainen, et al., 'Infant vitamin D supplementation and allergic conditions in adulthood: northern Finland birth cohort 1966', *Annals of the New York Academy of Sciences*, 2004, no. 1037, pp. 84–95.

Infant Feeding Advice, Australasian Society of Allergy and Immunology, http://www.allergy.org.au/images/stories/pospapers/

ascia_infantfeedingadvice_oct08.pdf, 2008.

Joffe, T. H., N. A. Simpson, 'Cesarean section and risk of asthma. The role of intrapartum antibiotics: a missing piece?', *Journal of Pediatrics*, 2009, no. 154, p. 154.

Johannsen, H. and S. L. Prescott, 'Practical prebiotics, probiotics and synbiotics for allergists: how useful are they?', *Clinical & Experimental Allergy*, 2009, no. 39, pp. 1801–14.

Kajosaari, M., U. M. Saarinen, 'Prophylaxis of atopic disease by six months' total solid food elimination. Evaluation of 135 exclusively breast-fed infants of atopic families', *Acta Paediatrica Scandinavia*, 1983, no. 72, pp. 411–4.

Kalliomäki, M., P. Kirjavainen, E. Eerola, P. Kero, S. Salminen, E. Isolauri, 'Distinct patterns of neonatal gut microflora in infants in whom atopy was and was not developing', *Journal of Allergy and Clinical Immunology*, 2001, no. 107, pp. 129–34.

Kalliomäki, M., S. Salminen, H. Arvilommi, P. Kero, P. Koskinen, E. Isolauri, 'Probiotics in primary prevention of atopic disease: a randomised placebo-controlled trial', *Lancet*, 2001, no. 357, pp. 1076–9.

Kalliomäki, M., S. Salminen, T. Poussa, H. Arvilommi, E. Isolauri, 'Probiotics and prevention of atopic disease: 4-year follow-up of a randomised placebo-controlled trial', *Lancet*, 2003, no. 361, pp. 1869–71.

Kalliomäki, M., S. Salminen, T. Poussa, E. Isolauri, 'Probiotics during the first 7 years of life: a cumulative risk reduction of eczema in a randomized, placebo-controlled trial', *Journal of Allergy and Clinical Immunology*, 2007, no. 119, pp. 1019–21.

Katelaris, C. H., J. E. Peake, 'Allergy and the skin: eczema and chronic urticaria', *Medical Journal of Australia*, 2006, no. 185, pp. 517–22.

Kim, K. Y., D. S. Kim, S. K. Lee, I. K. Lee, J. H. Kang, Y. S. Chang, et al., 'Association of low-dose exposure to persistent organic pollutants with global DNA hypomethylation in healthy koreans', *Environmental Health Perspectives*, 2010, no. 118, pp. 370–4.

Kjellman, N. I., 'Prediction and prevention of atopic allergy', *Allergy*, 1998, no. 53, pp. 67–71.

Knackstedt, M. K., E. Hamelmann, P. C. Arck, 'Mothers in stress: consequences for the offspring', *American Journal of Reproductive Immunology*, 2005, no. 54, pp. 63–9.

Kopp, M. V., I. Hennemuth, A. Heinzmann, R. Urbanek, 'Randomized, double-blind, placebo-controlled trial of probiotics for primary prevention: no clinical effects of *Lactobacillus* GG supplementation', *Pediatrics*, 2008, no. 121, pp. e850–6.

Koppelman, G. H., N. E. Reijmerink, O. Colin Stine, T. D. Howard, P. A. Whittaker, D. A. Meyers, et al., 'Association of a promoter polymorphism of the CD14 gene and atopy', *American Journal of Respiratory and Critical Care Medicine*, 2001, no. 163, pp.965–9.

Kramer, M.S., 'Maternal antigen avoidance during pregnancy for preventing atopic disease in infants of women at high risk', *Cochrane Database Systematic Review*, 2000, pp. 2.

Lack, G., 'Epidemiologic risks for food allergy', *Journal of Allergy and Clinical Immunology*, 2008, no. 121, pp. 1331-6.

Lai, C. K., R. Beasley, J. Crane, S. Foliaki, J. Shah, and S. Weiland, 'Global variation in the prevalence and severity of asthma symptoms: phase three of the International Study of Asthma and Allergies in Childhood (ISAAC)', *Thorax*, 2009, no. 64, pp. 476–83.

Lange, N. E., A. Litonjua, C. M. Hawrylowicz, S. Weiss, 'Vitamin D, the immune system and asthma', *Expert Review of Clinical Immunology*, 2009, no. 5, pp. 693–702.

Leung, D. Y. M., M. Boguniewicz, M. D. Howell, I. Nomura, Q.A. Hamid, 'New insights into atopic dermatitis', *Journal of Clinical Investigation*, 2004, no. 113, pp. 651–7.

Leung, T. F., N. L. Tang, Y. M. Sung, A. M. Li, G. W. Wong, I. H. Chan et al., 'The C-159T polymorphism in the CD14 promoter is associated with serum total IgE concentration in atopic Chinese children', *Pediatric Allergy and Immunology*, 2003, no. 14, pp. 255–60.

Lilja, G., A. Dannaeus, T. Foucard, V. Graff-Lonnevig, S. G. Johansson, H. Öman, 'Effects of maternal diet during late pregnancy and lactation on the development of atopic diseases in infants up to 18 months of age – in-vivo results', *Clinical & Experimental Allergy*, 1989, no. 19, pp. 473–9.

Litonjua, A. A., V. J. Carey, H. A. Burge, S. T. Weiss, D. R. Gold, 'Parental history and the risk for childhood asthma. Does mother confer more risk than father?' *American Journal of Respiratory and Critical Care Medicine*, 1998, no. 158, pp. 176–81.

Litonjua, A. A., S. T. Weiss, 'Is vitamin D deficiency to blame for the asthma epidemic?', *Journal of Allergy and Clinical Immunology*, 2007, no. 120, pp. 1031–5.

McGwin, G., J. Lienert, J. I. Kennedy, 'Formaldehyde exposure and asthma in children: a systematic review', *Environmental Health Perspectives*, 2010, no. 118, pp. 313–17.

McKeever, T. M., S. A. Lewis, C. Smith, J. Collins, H. Heatlie, M. Frischer, et al., 'Early exposure to infections and antibiotics and the incidence of allergic disease: a birth cohort study with the West Midlands General Practice Research Database', *Journal of Allergy and Clinical Immunology*, 2002, no. 109, pp. 43–50.

Marks, G. B., S. Mihrshahi, A. S. Kemp, E. R. Tovey, K. Webb, C. Almqvist et al., 'Prevention of asthma during the first 5 years of life: a randomized controlled trial', *Journal of Allergy and Clinical Immunology*, 2006, no. 118, pp. 53–61.

Martinez, F., A. Wright, L. Taussig, et al., 'Asthma and wheezing in the first six years of life', *New England Journal of Medicine*, 1995, no. 332, pp. 133–8.

Martino D., S. L. Prescott, 'Silent mysteries: epigenetic paradigms could hold the key to conquering the epidemic of allergy and immune disease', *Allergy*, 2010, vol. 65, no. 1, pp. 7–15.

Maslowski, K. M., A. T. Vieira, A. Ng, J. Kranich, F. Sierro, D. Yu, et al., 'Regulation of inflammatory responses by gut microbiota and chemoattractant receptor GPR43', *Nature*, 2009, no. 461, pp. 1282–6.

Metsala, J., A. Kilkkinen, M. Kaila, H. Tapanainen, T. Klaukka, M. Gissle, et al., 'Perinatal factors and the risk of asthma in childhood—a population-based register study in Finland', *American Journal of Epidemiology*, 2008, no. 168, pp. 170–8.

Miller, R. L., S. M. Ho, 'Environmental epigenetics and asthma: current concepts and call for studies', *American Journal of Respiratory and Critical Care Medicine*, 2008, no. 177, pp. 567–73.

Miyake, Y., S. Sasaki, K. Tanaka, Y. Hirota, 'Dairy food, calcium, and vitamin D intake in pregnancy and wheeze and eczema in infants', *European Respiratory Journal*, 2009.

Moller, C., H. Ahlstrom, K. A. Henricson, et al., 'Safety of nasal budesonide in the long-term treatment of children with perennial rhinitis', *Clinical & Experimental Allergy*, 2003, no. 33, pp. 816–22.

Möller, C., S. Dreborg, H. A. Ferdousi, S. Halken, A. Host, L. Jacobsen, et al., 'Pollen immunotherapy reduces the development of asthma in children with seasonal rhinoconjunctivitis (the PAT-study)', *Journal of Allergy and Clinical Immunology*, 2002, no. 109, pp. 251–6.

Morgan, J., P. Williams, F. Norris, C. M. Williams, M. Larkin, S. Hampton, 'Eczema and early solid feeding in preterm infants', *Archive of Disease in Childhood*, 2004, no. 89, pp. 309–14.

Moro, G, S. Arslanoglu, B. Stahl, J. Jelinek, U. Wahn, G. Boehm. 'A mixture of prebiotic oligosaccharides reduces the incidence of atopic dermatitis during the first six months of age', *Archive of Disease in Childhood*, 2006, no. 91, pp. 814–9.

Mosmann, T.R., R.L. Coffman, 'Heterogeneity of cytokine secretion patterns and functions of helper T cells', *Advanced Immunology*, 1989, no. 46, pp. 111–47.

Mullins R. J., 'Paediatric food allergy trends in a community-based specialist allergy practice, 1995–2006', *The Medical Journal of Australia*, 2007, no. 186, pp. 618–21.

Mullins, R. J., C. A. Camargo Jr., 'Shining a light on vitamin D and its impact on the developing immune system', *Clinical & Experimental Allergy*, 2011, no. 41, pp. 766–8.

Mullins, R. J., S. Clark, C. Katelaris, V. Smith, G, Solley, C. A. Camargo Jr., 'Season of birth and childhood food allergy in Australia', *Pediatric*

Allergy and Immunology, 2011, ePub.

Murr, C., K. Schroecksnadel, C. Winkler, M. Ledochowski, D. Fuchs, 'Antioxidants may increase the probability of developing allergic disease and asthma', *Medical Hypotheses*, 2005, no. 64, pp. 973–7.

Nakagomi, T., H. Itaya, T. Tominaga, M. Yamaka, S. Hisamatsu, O. Nagagomi, 'Is atopy increasing?', *Lancet*, 1994, vol. 341, pp. 121–2.

Ninan, T., G. Russell, 'Respiratory symptoms and atopy in Aberdeen school children: evidence from two surveys 25 years apart', *British Medical Journal*, 1992, vol. 304, pp. 873–75.

Noakes, P. S., J. Hale, R. Thomas, C. Lane, S. G. Devadason, S. L. Prescott, 'Maternal smoking is associated with impaired neonatal toll-like-receptor-mediated immune responses', *European Respiratory Journal*, 2006, no. 28, pp. 721–9.

Noakes, P. S., P. G. Holt, S. L. Prescott, 'Maternal smoking in pregnancy alters neonatal cytokine responses', *Allergy*, 2003, no. 58, pp. 1053–8.

Noakes. P. S., P. Taylor, S. Wilkinson, S. L. Prescott, 'The relationship between persistent organic pollutants in maternal and neonatal tissues and immune responses to allergens: A novel exploratory study', *Chemosphere*, 2006, no. 63, pp. 1304–11.

Norris, J. M., K. Barriga, E. J. Hoffenberg, I. Taki, D. Miao, J. E. Haas, et al., 'Risk of Celiac Disease Autoimmunity and Timing of Gluten Introduction in the Diet of Infants at Increased Risk of Disease', *JAMA*, 2005, no. 293, pp. 2343–51.

Nowak-Wegrzyn, A., H. A. Sampson, R. A. Wood, S. H. Sicherer, 'Food protein induced enterocolitis syndrome caused by solid food proteins', *Pediatrics*, 2003, no. 111, pp. 829–35.

Ober, C., A. Tsalenko, R. Parry, N. J. Cox, 'A second-generation genome-wide screen for asthma-susceptibility alleles in a founder population', *American Journal of Human Genetics*, 2000, no. 67, pp. 1154–62.

Oddy, W. H., N.H. de Klerk, P. D. Sly, P. G. Holt, 'The effects of respiratory infections, atopy, and breastfeeding on childhood asthma', *European Respiratory Journal*, 2002, no. 19, pp. 899–905.

Odhiambo, J. A., H. C. Williams, T. O. Clayton, C. F. Robertson,

M. I. Asher and the ISAAC Phase Three Study Group, 'Global map of eczema: Eczema symptoms in children from the International Study of Asthma and Allergies in Childhood (ISAAC) Phase Three', *Journal of Allergy and Clinical Immunology*, 2009, vol. 124, no. 6, pp. 1251–8.

Olsen, S. F., M. L. Osterdal, J. D. Salvig, L. M. Mortensen, D. Rytter, N. J. Secher, et al., 'Fish oil intake compared with olive oil intake in late pregnancy and asthma in the offspring: 16 years of registry-based follow-up from a randomized controlled trial', *American Journal of Clinical Nutrition*, 2008, no. 88, pp. 167–75.

Onufrak, S., J. Abramson, V. Vaccarino, 'Adult-onset asthma is associated with increased carotid atherosclerosis among women in the Atherosclerosis Risk in Communities (ARIC) study', *Atherosclerosis*, 2007, no. 195, pp. 129–37.

Osborn, D., J. Sinn, 'Formulas containing hydrolysed protein for prevention of allergy and food intolerance in infants', *Cochrane Database Systematic Review*, 2003, no. 4, CD003664.

——'Probiotics in infants for prevention of allergic disease and food hypersensitivity', *Cochrane Database Systematic Review*, 2007, no. 4, CD006475.

Osborne, N. J., J. J. Koplin, P. E. Martin, L. C. Gurrin, A. J. Lowe, M. C. Matheson, et al., 'Prevalence of challenge-proven IgE-mediated food allergy using population-based sampling and predetermined challenge criteria in infants', *Journal of Allergy and Clinical Immunology*, 2011, no. 127, pp. 668–76.

Ostblom, E., M. Wickman, M. van Hage, G. Lilja, 'Reported symptoms of food hypersensitivity and sensitization to common foods in 4-year-old children', *Acta Peadiatrica*, 2008, no. 97, pp. 85–90.

Osterballe, M., T. K. Hansen, C. G. Mortz, A. Host, C. Bindslev-Jensen, 'The prevalence of food hypersensitivity in an unselected population of children and adults', *Pediatric Allergy and Immunology*, 2005, no. 16, pp. 567–73.

Ownby, D. R., C. C. Johnson, E. L. Peterson, 'Exposure to dogs and cats in the first year of life and risk of allergic sensitization at 6 to 7 years of age', *JAMA*, 2002, no. 288, pp. 963–72.

Pajno, G. B., G Bearberio, F. de Luca, L. Morabito, S. Parmiani, 'Prevention of new sensitisations in asthmatic children monosensitised to house dust mite by specific immunotherapy. A six year follow-up study', *Clinical & Experimental Allergy*, 2001, no. 31, pp. 1392–7.

Palmer, D., M. Makrides, T. Sullivan, M. Gold, S. L. Prescott, R. J. Heddle, et al., 'Effect of n-3 docosahexaenoic acid (DHA) supplementation in pregnancy on infant allergies in the first year of life: a randomised controlled trial', forthcoming.

Peat, J., C. Salome, A. Woolcock, 'Factors associated with bronchial hyper-responsiveness in Australian adults and children', *European Respiratory Journal*, 1992, no. 5, pp. 921–9.

Peat, J., R. van-den-Berg, W. Green, C. Mellis, S. Leeder, A. Woolcock, 'Changing prevalence of asthma in Australian school children', *British Medical Journal*, 1994, no. 308, pp. 1591–96.

Perera, F., W. Y. Tang, J. Herbstman, D. Tang, L. Levin, R. Miller, et al., 'Relation of DNA methylation of 5'-CpG island of ACSL3 to transplacental exposure to airborne polycyclic aromatic hydrocarbons and childhood asthma', *PLoS One*, 2009, no. 4, pp. e4488.

Persky, V., J. Piorkowski, E. Hernandez, N. Chavez, C. Wagner-Cassanova, C. Vergara, et al., 'Prenatal exposure to acetaminophen and respiratory symptoms in the first year of life', *Annals of Allergy, Asthma & Immunology*, 2008, no. 101, pp. 271–8.

Platts-Mills, T. A., M. Perzanowski, J. A. Woodfolk, B. Lundbäck, 'Relevance of early or current pet ownership to the prevalence of allergic diseases', *Clinical & Experimental Allergy*, 2002, no. 32, p. 1259.

Ponsonby, A. L., T. Dwyer, A. Kemp, D. Couper, J. Cochrane, A. Carmichael, 'A prospective study of the association between home gas appliance use during infancy and subsequent dust mite sensitization and lung function in childhood', *Clinical & Experimental Allergy*, 2001, no. 31, pp. 1544–52.

Poole, J. A., K. Barriga, D. Y. M. Leung, D. R. Hoffman, G. Eisenbarth, M. Rewers, et al., 'Timing of Initial Exposure to Cereal Grains and the

Risk of Wheat Allergy', *Pediatrics*, 2006, vol. 117, no. 6, pp. 2175–82.

Prescott, S. L., 'Allergy: the price we pay for cleaner living?', *Annals of Allergy, Asthma & Immunology*, 2003, no. 90, pp. 64–70.

Prescott, S. L., K. A. Allen, 'Food Allergy: Riding the second wave of the allergy epidemic', *Paediatric Allergy and Immunology*, 2011, no. 22, pp. 155–60.

Prescott, S. L., B. Björkstén, 'Probiotics for the prevention or treatment of allergic diseases', *Journal of Allergy and Clinical Immunology*, 2007, no. 120, pp. 255–62.

Prescott, S. L., L. A. Breckler, C. S. Witt, L. Smith, J. A. Dunstan, F. T. Christiansen, 'Allergic women show reduced T helper type 1 alloresponses to fetal human leucocyte antigen mismatch during pregnancy', *Clinical & Experimental Allergy*, 2010, no. 159, pp. 65–72.

Prescott S. L., V. L. Clifton, 'Asthma and Pregnancy: emerging evidence of epigenetic interactions in utero', *Current Opinion in Allergy and Clinical Immunology*, 2009, vol. 9, no. 5, pp. 417–26.

Prescott, S. L., P. G. Holt, 'Abnormalities in cord blood mononuclear cytokine production as a predictor of later atopic disease in childhood' *Clinical & Experimental Allergy*, 1998, no. 28, pp. 1313–16.

Prescott, S. L., J. Irvine, J. A. Dunstan, C. Hii, A. Ferrante, 'Protein kinase-C zeta: a novel "protective" neonatal T cell marker that can be up-regulated by allergy prevention strategies', *Journal of Allergy and Clinical Immunology*, 2007, no. 120 pp. 200–6.

Prescott, S. L., M. Jenmalm, B. Björkstén, P. Holt, 'Effects of maternal allergen-specific IgG in cordblood on early postnatal development of allergen-specific T-cell immunity', *Allergy*, 2000, no. 55, pp. 470–5.

Prescott, S. L., P. Smith, M. L. K. Tang, D. J. Palmer, J. Sinn, S. J. Huntley, et al., 'The importance of early complementary feeding in the development of oral tolerance: concerns and controversies', *Pediatric Allergy and Immunology*, 2008, vol. 19, no. 5, pp. 375–80.

Prescott, S. L., C. Macaubas, B. Holt, T. Smallacombe, R. Loh, P. Sly, et al., 'Transplacental priming of the human immune system to environmental allergens: universal skewing of initial T-cell responses towards Th-2 cytokine profile', *Journal of Immunology*, 1998, no. 160, pp. 4730–7.

——'Development of allergen-specific T-cell memory in atopic and normal children', *Lancet*, 1999, vol. 353, no. 9148, pp. 196–200.

——'Reciprocal age-related patterns of allergen-specific T-cell immunity in normal vs. atopic infants', *Clinical & Experimental Allergy*, 1998, no. 28, Suppl 5, pp. 39–44.

Prescott, S. L., M. L. Tang, 'The Australasian Society of Clinical Immunology and Allergy position statement: summary of allergy prevention in children', *Medical Journal of Australia*, 2005, no. 182, pp. 464–7.

Prescott, S. L., M. Tang, B. Björkstén, 'Primary allergy prevention in children 2007: a revised summary of the Australasian Society of Clinical Immunology and Allergy Position Statement', *Medical Journal of Australia*, 2007

Raby, B. A., R. Lazarus, E. K. Silverman, S. Lake, C. Lange, M. Wjst et al., 'Association of vitamin D receptor gene polymorphisms with childhood and adult asthma', *American Journal of Respiratory and Critical Care Medicine*, 2004, no. 170, pp. 1057–65.

Rebordosa, C., M. Kogevinas, H. T. Sorensen, J. Olsen, 'Pre-natal exposure to paracetamol and risk of wheezing and asthma in children: a birth cohort study', *International Journal of Epidemiology*, 2008, no. 37, pp. 583–90.

Reichrtova, E., P. Ciznar, V. Prachar, L. Palkovicova, M. Veningerova, 'Cord serum immunoglobulin E related to the environmental contamination of human placentas with organochlorine compounds', *Environmental Health Perspectives*, 1999, no. 107, pp. 895–9.

Renz, H., E. von Mutius, P. Brandtzaeg, W. O. Cookson, I. B. Autenrieth, and D. Haller, 'Gene-environment interactions in chronic inflammatory disease', *Nature Immunology*, 2011, no. 1, pp.273–7.

Robertson, C., M. Dalton, J. Peat, M. Haby, A. Bauman, J. Kennedy, et al., 'Asthma and other atopic diseases in Australian children (Australian arm of the International Study of Asthma and Allergy in Childhood)',

The Medical Journal of Australia, 1998, no. 168, pp. 434–8.

Robertson, C. F., M. F. Roberts, J. H. Kappers, 'Asthma prevalence in Melbourne schoolchildren: have we reached the peak?', *The Medical Journal of Australia*, 2004, no. 180, pp. 273–6.

Rowe, J., C. Macaubas, T. Monger, B. J. Holt, J. Harvey, J. T. Poolman et al., 'Heterogeneity in diphtheria-tetanus-acellular pertussis vaccine-specific cellular immunity during infancy: relationship to variations in the kinetics of postnatal maturation of systemic th1 function', *Journal of Infectious Diseases*, 2001, no. 184, pp. 80–8.

Salam, M. T., Y. F. Li, B. Langholz, F. D. Gilliland, 'Maternal fish consumption during pregnancy and risk of early childhood asthma', *Journal of Asthma*, 2005, no. 42, pp. 513–8.

Sampson, H. A., 'Food allergy', *Journal of Allergy and Clinical Immunology*, 2003, no. 111, pp. S540–7.

Sausenthaler, S., S. Koletzko, B. Schaaf, I. Lehmann, M. Borte, O. Herbarth, et al., 'Maternal diet during pregnancy in relation to eczema and allergic sensitization in the offspring at 2 y of age', *American Journal of Clinical Nutrition*, 2007, no. 85, p. 530.

Savage, J. H., E. C. Matsui, J. M. Skripak, R. A. Wood, 'The natural history of egg allergy', *Journal of Allergy and Clinical Immunology*, 2007, no. 120, pp. 1413–7.

Schaub, B., J. Liu, S. Hoppler, S. Haug, C. Sattler, A. Lluis, et al., 'Impairment of T-regulatory cells in cord blood of atopic mothers', *Journal of Allergy and Clinical Immunology*, 2008, no. 121, pp. 1491–9, 9 e1–13.

Schaub, B., J. Liu, S. Hoppler, I. Schleich, J. Huehn, S. Olek, et al., 'Maternal farm exposure modulates neonatal immune mechanisms through regulatory T cells', *Journal of Allergy and Clinical Immunology*, 2009, no. 123, pp. 774–82 e5.

Schofield, A. T., 'A case of egg poisoning,' *Lancet*, 1908, no. 1, p. 716.

Scholtens, P. A., P. Alliet, M. Raes, M. S. Alles, H. Kroes, G. Boehm, et al., 'Fecal secretory immunoglobulin A is increased in healthy infants who receive a formula with short-chain galacto-oligosaccharides and long-chain fructo-oligosaccharides', *Journal of Nutrition*, 2008, no. 138, pp. 1141–7.

Schouten, B., B. C. van Esch, G. A. Hofman, S. A. van Doorn, J. Knol, A. J. Nauta, et al., 'Cow milk allergy symptoms are reduced in mice fed dietary synbiotics during oral sensitization with whey', *Journal of Nutrition*, 2009, no. 139, pp. 1398–403

Sepp, E., K. Julge, M. Vasar, P. Naaber, B. Björkstén, M. Mikelsaar, 'Intestinal microflora of Estonian and Swedish infants', *Acta Paediatrica*, 1997, no. 86, pp. 956–61.

Shaheen, S. O., 'Prenatal nutrition and asthma: hope or hype?', *Thorax*, 2008, no. 63, pp. 483–5.

Shaheen, S. O., R. B. Newson, A. Sherriff, A. J. Henderson, J. E. Heron, P. G. Burney, et al., Paracetamol use in pregnancy and wheezing in early childhood', *Thorax*, 2002, no. 57, pp. 958–63.

Sicherer, S. H., A. Munoz-Furlong, J. H. Godbold, H. A. Sampson, 'US prevalence of self-reported peanut, tree nut, and sesame allergy: 11-year follow-up', *Journal of Allergy and Clinical Immunology*, forthcoming.

Sicherer, S. H., H. A. Sampson, 'Food allergy', *Journal of Allergy and Clinical Immunology*, 2006, no. 117, pp. S470–5.

Sigurs, N., R. Bjarnason, F. Sigurbergsson, B. Kjellman, B. Björkstén, 'Asthma and immunoglobulin E antibodies after respiratory syncytial virus bronchiolitis: a prospective cohort study with matched controls', *Pediatrics*, 1995, no. 95, pp. 500–5.

Sigurs, N., G. Hattevig, B. Kjellman, 'Maternal avoidance of eggs, cow's milk, and fish during lactation: effect on allergic manifestations, skin-prick tests, and specific IgE antibodies in children at age 4 years', *Pediatrics*, 1992, no. 89, pp. 735–9.

Simpson, A., S. L. John, F. Jury, R. Niven, A. Woodcock, W. E. Ollier et al., 'Endotoxin exposure, CD14, and allergic disease: an interaction between genes and the environment', *American Journal of Respiratory and Critical Care Medicine*, 2006, no. 174, pp. 386–92.

Simpson, S. J., G. A. Sword, 'Phase polyphenism in locusts: Mechanisms, population consequences, adaptive significance and evolution', in *Phenotypic Plasticity of Insects: Mechanisms and Consequences*, Ed. D. Whitman, and T. Ananthakrishnan, Plymouth, Science Publishers, Inc., 2009, pp. 147–90.

Sjogren, Y. M., M. C. Jenmalm, M. F. Bottcher, B. Björkstén, E. Sverremark-Ekstrom, 'Altered early infant gut microbiota in children developing allergy up to 5 years of age', *Clinical & Experimental Allergy*, 2009, no. 39, pp. 518–26.

Skripak, J. M., E. C. Matsui, K. Mudd, R. A. Wood, 'The natural history of IgE-mediated cow's milk allergy', *Journal of Allergy and Clinical Immunology*, 2007, no. 120, pp. 1172–7.

Smith, M., M. R. Tourigny, P. Noakes, C. A. Thornton, M. K. Tulic, S. L. Prescott, 'Children with egg allergy have evidence of reduced neonatal CD4(+)CD25(+)CD127(lo/-) regulatory T cell function', *Journal of Allergy and Clinical Immunology*, 2008, no. 121, pp. 1460–6, 6 e1–7.

Soni, A., 'Allergic Rhinitis: Trends in Use and Expenditures, 2000 and 2005', *Medical Expenditure Panel Survey*, Center for Financing, Access, and Cost Trends, Agency for Healthcare Research and Quality, Rockville, MD, 2008.

Strachan, D. P., 'Hay fever, hygiene, and household size', *British Medical Journal*, 1989, no. 299, pp. 1259–60.

——'Family size, infection and atopy: the first decade of the "hygiene hypothesis"', *Thorax*, 2000, no. 55, Suppl 1, pp. S2–10.

Sudo, N., S. Sawamura, K. Tanaka, Y. Aiba, C. Kubo, Y. Koga, 'The requirement of intestinal bacterial flora for the development of an IgE production system fully susceptible to oral tolerance induction', *Journal of Immunology*, 1997, no. 159, pp. 1739–45.

Suissa, S., T. Assimes, P. Brassard, P. Ernst, 'Inhaled corticosteroid use in asthma and the prevention of myocardial infarction', *American Journal of Medicine*, 2003, no. 115, pp. 377–81.

Tan, P. H., P. Sagoo, C. Chan, J. B. Yates, J. Campbell, S. C. Beutelspacher, et al., 'Inhibition of NF-kappa B and oxidative pathways in human dendritic cells by antioxidative vitamins generates regulatory T cells',

Journal of Immunology, 2005, no. 174, pp. 7633–44.

Tang, M. L. K., A. S. Kemp, J. Thorburn, D. Hill, 'Reduced interferon gamma secretion in neonates and subsequent atopy', *Lancet*, 1994, no. 344, pp. 983–5.

Taylor, A. L., J. A. Dunstan, S. L. Prescott, 'Probiotic supplementation for the first 6 months of life fails to reduce the risk of atopic dermatitis and increases the risk of allergen sensitization in high-risk children: a randomized controlled trial', *Journal of Allergy and Clinical Immunology*, 2007, no. 119, pp. 184–91.

Thavagnanam, S., J. Fleming, A. Bromley, M. D. Shields, C. R. Cardwell, 'A meta-analysis of the association between Caesarean section and childhood asthma', *Clinical & Experimental Allergy*, 2008, no. 38, pp. 629–33.

'The economic impact of allergic disease in Australia: not to be sneezed at', *Report by Access Economics Pty Ltd for the Australasian Society of Clinical Immunology and Allergy* (ASCIA), 2007.

Thien, F. C. K., 'Drug hypersensitivity', *Medical Journal of Australia*, 2006, no. 185, pp. 333–8.

Tollanes, M. C., D. Moster, A. K. Daltveit, L. M. Irgens, 'Cesarean section and risk of severe childhood asthma: a population-based cohort study', *Journal of Pediatrics*, 2008, no. 153, pp. 112–6.

Tulic, M., A. Forsberg, M. Hodder, S. McCarthy, D. Martino, N. de Vaz N, et al., 'Differences in the developmental trajectory of innate microbial responses in atopic and normal children: new insights into immune ontogeny', *Journal of Allergy and Clinical Immunology*, 2011, no. 127, no. 2, pp.:470–8.

Utsugi, M., K. Dobashi, T. Ishizuka, K. Endou, J. Hamuro, Y. Murata, et al., 'c-Jun N-terminal kinase negatively regulates lipopolysaccharide-induced IL-12 production in human macrophages: role of mitogen-activated protein kinase in glutathione redox regulation of IL-12 production', *Journal of Immunology*, 2003, vol. 171, no. 2, pp. 628–35.

van Hoffen, E., B. Ruiter, J. Faber, L. M'Rabet, E. F. Knol, B. Stahl, et al., 'A specific mixture of short-chain galacto-oligosaccharides and long-chain fructo-oligosaccharides induces a beneficial immuno-globulin profile in infants at high risk for allergy', *Allergy*, 2009, no. 64, pp. 484–7.

Varshney, P., S. M. Jones, A. M. Scurlock, T. T. Perry, A. Kemper, P. Steele, et al., 'A randomized controlled study of peanut oral immu-notherapy: clinical desensitization and modulation of the allergic response', *Journal of Allergy and Clinical Immunology*, 2011, no. 127, pp. 654–60.

Vassallo, M. F., A. Banerji, S. A. Rudders, S. Clark, R. J. Mullins, C. A. Camargo Jr., 'Season of birth and food allergy in children', *Annals of Allergy, Asthma and Immunology*, 2010, no. 104, pp. 307–13.

Venter, C., B. Pereira, J. Grundy, C. B. Clayton, S. H. Arshad, T. Dean, 'Prevalence of sensitization reported and objectively assessed food hypersensitivity amongst six-year-old children: a population-based study', *Pediatric Allergy and Immunology*, 2006, no. 17, pp. 356–63.

von Berg, A., B. Filipiak-Pittroff, U. Kramer, E. Link, C. Bollrath, I. Brockow, et al., 'Preventive effect of hydrolyzed infant formulas persists until age 6 years: Long-term results from the German Infant Nutritional Intervention Study (GINI)', *Journal of Allergy and Clinical Immunology*, 2008, no. 121, pp. 1442–7.

von Mutius, E., F. D. Martinez, C. Fritzsch, T. Nicolai, G. Roell, H. H. Thiemann, 'Prevalence of asthma and atopy in two areas of West and East Germany,' *American Journal of Respiratory and Critical Care Medicine*, 1994, no. 149, pp. 358–64.

von Mutius, E., S. K. Weiland, C. Fritzsch, H. Duhme, U. Keil, 'Increasing prevalence of hay fever and atopy among children in Leipzig, East Germany', *Lancet*, 1998, no. 351, pp. 862–6.

Wadhwa, P. D., C. Busd, S. Entringer, J. M. Swanson, 'Developmental origins of health and disease: brief history of the approach and current focus on epigenetic mechanisms', *Seminars in Reproductive Medicine*, 2009, no. 27, pp. 358–68.

Walls, R. S., R. J. Heddle, M. L. K. Tang, B. J. Basger, G. O. Solley, G.

T. Yeo, 'Optimising the management of allergic rhinitis: an Australian perspective', *Medical Journal of Australia*, 2005, no. 182, pp. 28–33.

Wegmann, T. G., H. Lin, L. Guilbert, T. R. Mosmann, 'Bidirectional cytokine interactions in the maternal-fetal relationship: is successful pregnancy a Th2 phenomenon?', *Immunology Today*, 1993, vol. 14, no. 7, pp. 353–6.

Weiner, J. M., 'Allergen injection immunotherapy', *Medical Journal of Australia*, 2006, vol. 185, no.4, p. 234.

Weiss, S. T., 'Bacterial components plus vitamin D: The ultimate solution to the asthma (autoimmune disease) epidemic?', *Journal of Allergy and Clinical Immunology*, 2011, no. 127, pp. 1128–30.

Weiss, S. T., A. A. Litonjua, 'The in utero effects of maternal vitamin D deficiency: how it results in asthma and other chronic diseases', *American Journal of Respiratory and Critical Care Medicine*, 2011, no. 183, pp. 1286–7.

West, C. E., D. Videky, S. L. Prescott, 'Role of diet in the development of immune tolerance in the context of allergic disease', *Current Opinion in Pediatrics*, 2010, no. 2, pp. 635–41.

Whitrow, M. J., V. M. Moore, A. R. Rumbold, M. J. Davies, 'Effect of supplemental folic acid in pregnancy on childhood asthma: a prospective birth cohort study', *American Journal of Epidemiology*, 2009, no. 170, pp. 1486–93.

Wildhaber, J. H., S. G. Devadason, M. J. Hayden, E. Eber, Q. A. Summers, P. N. LeSouef, 'Aerosol delivery to wheezy infants: a comparison between a nebulizer and two small volume spacers', *Pediatric Pulmonology*, 1997, no. 23, pp. 212–16.

Wills-Karp, M., J. Santeliz, C. L. Karp, 'The germless theory of allergic disease: revisiting the hygiene hypothesis', *National Review of Immunology*, 2001, no. 1, pp. 69–75.

Wilson, A. C., J. S. Forsyth, S. A. Greene, L. Irvine, C. Hau, P. W. Howie, 'Relation of infant diet to childhood health: seven year follow up of cohort of children in Dundee infant feeding study', *BMJ*, 1998, no. 316, pp. 21–5.

Wjst, M., 'The vitamin D slant on allergy', *Pediatric Allergy and Immunology*, 2006, no. 17, pp. 477–83.

Wolkoff, P., G. D. Nielsen, 'Non-cancer effects of formaldehyde and relevance for setting an indoor air guideline', *Environment International*, 2010.

Woodcock, A., L. A. Lowe, C. S. Murray, B. M. Simpson, S. D. Pipis, P. Kissen et al., 'Early life environmental control: effect on symptoms, sensitization, and lung function at age 3 years', *American Journal of Respiratory and Critical Care Medicine*, 2004, no. 170, pp. 433–9.

World Allergy Organization (WAO), *White Book on Allergy*, Ruby Pawankar, Giorgio Walter Canonica, Stephen T. Holgate and Richard F. Lockey (eds), Milwaukee, Wisconsin, World Allergy Organization (www.worldallergy.org), 2011.

World Health Organisation, 'Global surveillance, prevention and control of chronic respiratory diseases: a comprehensive approach', World Health Organisation, 2007.

Zeiger, R., S. Heller, M. Mellon, J. Halsey, R. Hamburger, H. Sampson, 'Genetic and environmental factors affecting the development of atopy through age 4 in children with atopic parents: a prospective radomised study of food allergen avoidance', *Pediatric Allergy and Immunology*, 1992, no.3, pp. 110–27.

Zutavern, A., I. Brockow, B. Schaaf, G. Bolte, A. von Berg, U. Diez, et al., 'Timing of solid food introduction in relation to atopic dermatitis and atopic sensitization: results from a prospective birth cohort study', *Pediatrics*, 2006, no. 117, pp. 401–11.

Zutavern, A., E. von Mutius, J. Harris, P. Mills, S. Moffat, C. White, et al., 'The introduction of solids in relation to asthma and eczema', *Archive of Diseases of Childhood*, 2004, no. 89, pp. 303–8.